Dr Nick Fuller is a leading obesity researcher in Australia and has been running the clinical research program at the Boden Institute, Charles Perkins Centre, at the University of Sydney for the past decade. He has helped hundreds of people with their weight-loss and lifestyle journeys and investigated a broad range of topics, including dietary and exercise programs, appetite hormones, commercial programs, complementary and conventional medicines, medical devices and weight-loss surgery. He holds a doctorate on the efficacy and cost-effectiveness of different obesity weight-loss treatments, as well as degrees in exercise physiology, nutrition and dietetics.

interval
WEIGHT
LOSS

Dr Nick Fuller

EBURY
PRESS

An Ebury Press book
Published by Penguin Random House Australia Pty Ltd
Level 3, 100 Pacific Highway, North Sydney NSW 2060
www.penguin.com.au

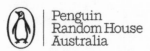 Penguin
Random House
Australia

First published by Ebury Press in 2017

Copyright © Nicholas Fuller, 2017

The moral right of the author has been asserted.

Addresses for the Penguin Random House group of companies can be found at global.penguinrandomhouse.com/offices.

National Library of Australia
Cataloguing-in-Publication entry

Fuller, Nick, author
Interval weight loss / Nick Fuller

ISBN 978 0 14378 5 361 (paperback)

Weight loss
Body diet
Reducing diets – Recipes

Author photograph by David Griffiths
Cover illustration courtesy of Shutterstock
Cover design by Alex Ross © Penguin Random House Australia Pty Ltd
Internal design by Midland Typesetters, Australia
Typeset in 13.5/18 pt Adobe Garamond Pro by Midland Typesetters, Australia
Printed in Australia by Griffin Press, an accredited ISO AS/NZS 14001:2004
Environmental Management System printer

Penguin Random House Australia uses papers that are natural, renewable and recyclable products and made from wood grown in sustainable forests. The logging and manufacturing processes are expected to conform to the environmental regulations of the country of origin.

'If you always do what you've always done,
you'll always get what you've always got.'

Henry Ford

This book is for you, Dad.

You were a well-loved and influential figure. I will forever be grateful to you and Mum for your hard work, devotion and self-sacrifice. You have inspired me to put my thoughts into writing, to help others on their journeys, and to chase my dreams.

You will forever be in my thoughts.

CONTENTS

PROLOGUE

From an early age I had a passion for nutrition, stemming from the influence of my father, who had a keen interest in health and exercise. As an adult I turned this passion into a vocation and have spent the past ten years researching obesity and running clinical trials. I have also worked in industry and corporate settings, helping people to lose weight. In that time I have witnessed firsthand my patients' confusion over which diet they should follow and frustration at their inability to lose weight. Some of those who come to me have spent years trying to slim down and get healthy. Little wonder they are confused when there are so many bad books on nutrition written by unqualified people and filled with misinformation on 'diets'.

This book is aimed at clearing up the misconceptions and confusion, and to arm you with the latest science so as to lose weight and keep it off, using my interval weight-loss approach. It's easy to follow, won't break the bank and is based on scientific research and my experiences with hundreds of patients. This is *not* a book about a diet – it is factual information that you can use to trick your body into losing weight, and to create a plan that will bring structure and routine into your life for a healthier you. So, if you've tried every diet under the sun and still put on weight, give it a go – you have nothing to lose but the kilos.

PART 1

CHAPTER 1

THE PROBLEM
WITH FAD DIETS

'Failure isn't fatal, but failure to
change might be.' – *John Wooden*

Approximately two in three adults are overweight or
obese in Australia[1], and in most countries the problem
is only escalating, making it a global epidemic. A large shift
in technological advancement means that we now live in an
environment that challenges us to lead a healthy lifestyle.

Back in the 1970s we used to engage in more leisure
activities, walk everywhere, and often had more physical
jobs. We would play in the park with our children and
visit friends, instead of spending time on mobile phones,
video games and computers. By contrast, nowadays we are
time-poor, we work longer hours, and more is expected
of us both at home and at work. Work–life balance is

rare as we devote less and less time to our health. As a result, we simply don't move enough, and we frequently consume high-energy convenience foods, which results in weight gain.

What has this meant for us? Well, we now live in a world where fitness centres and gyms are popping up on every corner, and every week someone else is publishing the next weight-loss diet that will solve everyone's problems. But rather than solve anything, things have only got worse – much worse. Despite the fact that most of all known modern diets were invented from the 1980s onwards, obesity rates since then have actually trebled![2] Clearly, diets have done nothing to curb the obesity epidemic. If anything, it could be argued that diets have contributed to the rise of the very thing they claim to diminish: we are dieting ourselves to obesity.

In order to examine how this contradiction is possible, let's consider a patient of mine. Jennifer, a 29-year-old female, is a comfortable 68 kilograms. At 169 centimetres tall and with a body fat of 28 per cent she would be considered in the healthy weight range. Jennifer is going on a beach holiday to Hawaii in six weeks and her stated goal is to get her weight down to 62 kilos by the time she leaves. This equates to a total body weight reduction of approximately 9 per cent. The good news is that through a series of detox teas, vegetable soups and a total ban of all sweets, Jennifer is successful at hitting her desired weight for the Hawaii trip. She has a fabulous holiday and meets a nice new bloke from Toowoomba.

So what's the problem? I hear you say. In isolation, nothing! Except something happens over the next few months after Jennifer's return. Her body's innate response kicks in and it feels compelled to go back to its pre-defined pre-holiday weight. For every action there is an equal and opposite reaction. But, listen up, Jennifer does not return to 68 kilos. Due to the stress she has imposed on her body by her most recent diet, not to mention the many other diets she has been on previously, her body not only climbs back to its original weight, it blasts through 68 kilos like a Sunday morning cyclist whipping past you in canary yellow Lycra. Six months after the famous holiday where Jennifer met Mr Toowoomba, she has become worried that she's become 'fat'. 'How did this happen?' she asks herself while looking back at the holiday pictures. Good question, Jennifer!

The diet trap

Jennifer's question is a common one, and the answer is that dieting has resulted in her body going into a state of starvation due to severe energy and nutrient restriction. Her energy and nutritional intake were so low, and her diet so poor that her body in essence began to slow, or shut down metabolically, to hold onto its reserves in response to her weighing less. Accompanying this innate response to energy restriction was an increase in her appetite hormone signalling to her brain to tell her to eat more.

Research has shown that these appetite hormone levels remain elevated above normal a year after finishing a reduced-energy weight-loss diet.[3] What does that mean? It means that Jennifer's body is still signalling to her to eat more so that she can bounce back to her starting weight.

You might be saying to yourself, 'I'm not like Jennifer. Diets work for me,' and that may well be true the first time you go on a diet. The first time you follow one, you will lose weight (and it doesn't matter what the diet is), and you may keep it off for a while. But if you come off the diet, your weight is likely to rebound to where it was – if not a couple of kilograms higher than where you started, as was the case with Jennifer. The next time it will be harder to lose as much weight; and the time after that, even harder. As a result, your body weight will reset at a higher starting point each time you diet.

The comfort zone

The reason the scales keep going up is because we are tuned to a set body weight – a weight that the body feels most comfortable being. When you take your body out of that comfort zone through dieting or a reduction in energy intake, your body works to counteract the weight loss, and in a state of stress the body's innate response will be to store rather than offload weight. This is part of the fight or flight response (in this instance, the energy restriction is the acute stress our body is responding to) and is core to the survival of the human species. This weight regain comes with a greater initial increase in fat mass. However, our body weight will often keep going up until our muscle mass stores are restored and what you end up with is a body that has a little extra fat storage to survive the next 'starvation' (otherwise known as a diet) it has learned it needs to prepare for.

For those with lower initial body weights, it is often muscle mass that is lost when they diet and consequently these people suffer a larger weight regain until the muscle mass is restored to the baseline level. This increase in fat mass and then muscle mass (which is slower to regain) then puts you at a higher starting point than when you began. You are in essence dieting yourself fatter and fatter. As I'll explain later our focus should not, in fact, be on dieting at all and the very word 'diet' is one that I dislike enormously.

Fad diets

Most diets are not realistic weight-loss options, as they are not nutritionally balanced and therefore detrimental to your health long term. For example, the Palaeolithic

(Palaeo) diet is based on the principle that we should be eating the foods our ancestors ate because our gene pool has changed very little over all this time. However, many of the foods our hunter-gatherer ancestors ate do not even exist today – most modern crops and animals differ drastically from those of our ancestors' time, not just because of advances in technology but also due to natural selection. As a consequence our modern equivalents have different nutritional properties. For example, broccoli and kale didn't exist and instead derived from the ancient species *Brassica oleracea*.

Our evolution has meant that our ancestors simply wouldn't have survived in the modern world. The development of our brain size means that we require far more carbohydrate to match the glucose supply needed for the brain. As well as this, our ancestors' diets were lacking in essential nutrition (for example, fibre and calcium) and consequently they had poor bone and dental health and very short lifespans. They certainly could have been better off following a modern, balanced and nutritious diet, if accompanied by the same level of activity they were doing.

Furthermore, agricultural development, which the Palaeo diet condemns, started to take place thousands of years ago. And food processing – one of the biggest taboos of the diet – is not new either. For example, the origins of the hamburger – which has become one of the biggest scapegoats for the rise in obesity – dates back as far as 50 B.C. in China. So, what people consider western-ised foods, or foods making us 'fat', have in essence been around for a very long time. I'm not suggesting that you rush out to McDonald's and eat your body weight in Big Macs – far from it. My point here is simply that agriculture and food processing are not new, and definitely not the sole reasons for the rise in the number of overweight and obese people in the world, as many diets and celebrity 'experts' proclaim.

Setting yourself up for failure

Following the newest diet, whether it be the Palaeo diet, the lemon detox diet, the vegetable soup diet, the cabbage soup diet, the liver cleansing diet, the master cleanse diet, the Atkins diet, or even the onion diet (the list goes on and on), is the last thing you should be doing. These fad diets are just that – fads! And some diets are backed by claims that are not proven and that are false or misleading, propagated by people who are not qualified health professionals and whose suggestions are not backed by scientific literature.

Some of the companies espousing diets even have a vested interest in you not losing weight in the long term: they want you to buy more of the products accompanying their diets. It is in their interests to show you some quick results (confirmation of success) and then let you think that it is your fault when you put the weight back on, so that you will go and buy their next book/DVD, or whatever it is they are selling.

You are being set up to fail and to have a bigger weight problem in the future. As with the example of Jennifer, every time you lose weight on these diets, you are making it harder to keep the weight off long term. I have seen this time and time again with hundreds of my patients. I have met many people who are so desperate to do something about their body weight that they are willing to try anything.

Max, a 51-year-old male, weighed 106 kilograms when I met him, and at 183 centimetres tall was classified as obese. He weighed approximately 80 kilograms throughout most of his young-adult years; however, during his early 30s his life changed significantly. He took on a more senior employment role, got married and had children. His weight began to increase ever so slightly, which was enough for him to do something about it.

Instead of adopting the healthy principles he had always followed in his earlier years, he thought the easiest approach would be to lose weight through dieting. He went through the same process as Jennifer. Like her, he lost weight, but then regained it over time to the point where he was finding it hard to run around after his children.

Not to be deterred, he continued this dieting cycle each year, only making matters worse, and his weight continued to go up, spiralling out of control. By this stage he was beginning to panic, and to follow any new diet that hit the shelves or that he found on the internet, which only compounded his problem. It took a while to convince Max that dieting was not a sensible approach, but eventually he conceded that, since none of the diets he was following was working for him, maybe it was time to listen to a bona fide expert.

With my Interval Weight Loss plan, we quickly got his lifestyle back on track, and a healthy weight loss was achieved and maintained, much to his relief and the delight of his wife and children.

The first thing I'd like you to take from this example is that you must not go on the next celebrity or fad diet that hits the shelves. Ideally, though, I'd also like you to go a step further and eliminate the word 'diet' from your vocabulary. By doing those two very simple things, you are already going a long way to succeeding in your lifestyle and weight-loss journey.

There are, of course, weight-loss books that are better than others, and that have been written by qualified health professionals. They're not really diets per se, but rather holistic dietary plans, and teach the core principles of healthy eating and nutrition, such as those developed by leading scientific organisations like the Commonwealth Science and Industrial Research Organisation (CSIRO).

The CSIRO food plan has received some criticism for providing less then 40 per cent of energy from carbohydrates (which I believe is at the low end of ideal), but at least it acknowledges the importance of carbohydrates (especially the refined, processed type). However, in my opinion there is no need to restrict carbohydrate to such low levels, as there is no conclusive evidence to show a greater benefit long term. Also, crucially, the CSIRO food plan does not teach you how to reprogram your body, which I'll explain in the following chapters.

Then there are commercial weight-loss programs, such as Weight Watchers, which I have personally been involved in conducting clinical trials on. This type of commercial program is backed by scientific literature and teaches the principles of healthy eating via both a face-to-face group approach and the internet, significantly bringing down the cost to the consumer.

Lastly, there are scientifically proven cultural-eating patterns, such as the Mediterranean food plan, which are backed by a low prevalence, among those following it, of metabolic disorders or disease; specifically cardiovascular (heart) disease. The Mediterranean food plan includes heart-healthy foods rich in 'good' fats (fish, nuts and olive oil) and antioxidant-rich items such as red wine. It is a great non-fad, non-commercialised cultural eating plan that can be followed by anyone. As research has shown, fat is not the devil in all of this, and including plenty of good fats goes a long way to achieving a healthy lifestyle and your ideal weight. Again, though, as with any food plan, you will need to learn to reprogram your body, so read on for advice on how to do this. It's the key to your success.

Let's begin!

CHAPTER 2

REPROGRAMMING YOUR SET BODY WEIGHT

'The secret of change is to focus all of
your energy not on fighting the old but on
building the new.' – *Socrates*

As I've explained in the previous chapter, we are all
tuned to a set body weight. Our body weight is regulated via feedback that controls energy intake and energy
expenditure, resulting in the body protecting its level of
fat when too much food is consumed or too little activity
performed (i.e. when energy balance is disturbed). In the
academic world there have been several models proposed
and much debate as to how this regulation might take
place. However, regardless of how body weight regulation occurs, what seems certain is that there is a set body
weight that our body protects.

Yo-yoing weight

Your body does all it can to hold onto its reserves, and a person's metabolism (how much energy we burn at rest) will lower when put under stress – for example, under a period of significantly reduced food intake.

As I've said, crash dieting wreaks mayhem with your metabolism and body composition in a way that will see your weight decrease and increase in a cyclic fashion, with the trend not going down over time but up. Sure, there are some nutritionally balanced meal-replacement diets out there, but these are for specific medical purposes and do not represent sustainable long-term weight maintenance for the average person. If you want to lose weight and keep it off, meal replacements are not for you.

Preserving your metabolic rate

This book is about preventing any associated decrease in metabolism and reduction in muscle mass and consequent weight regain from dieting. Interval Weight Loss is instead focused on doing all it can to preserve or increase the amount of energy you burn at rest. It is not a traditional slow versus fast weight-loss approach, which results in the same amount of weight regain over a longer term three-year follow-up period[4] whatever approach you try. This plan is focused on minimising any loss of lean muscle mass associated with weight loss, and increase in appetite hormones associated with a large deficit in energy intake. We know that weight regain is driven by muscle mass and appetite regulating hormones, but one of the biggest challenges is that weight regain is often associated with a larger gain in fat mass as opposed to muscle mass. This is an unfavourable situation to be in, as muscle mass is metabolically active, meaning it burns more energy at rest than does fat. We'll learn more about this later, in Chapter 6, 'Exercise and rest'.

Set point

It's important to get the body outside of its normal comfort zone to achieve success and set you up for long-term weight-loss maintenance. This means you need to work towards redefining your set body weight over a gradual period. This is done by an Interval Weight Loss approach, by which I mean a period of weight loss followed by a period of weight maintenance. It has absolutely no fasting or dieting component, but instead relies on small changes to your nutritional intake and physical activity level, and closely monitoring your body weight on the scales. You might set a goal of a 2 kilogram weight loss over the first month, with your goal to maintain it over the second month, before then aiming for another 2 kilogram weight loss during the third month (more on how to do this in the next chapter), and then again maintaining it during the fourth month, and so on. This approach is in effect reprogramming your body weight to a new 'set point' and must be done gradually.

Tricking your body

You need to do all you can to prevent your weight from bouncing back to where you started and really convince your body that a 2 kilogram weight loss is your new 'set point'. I would recommend aiming for 1 to 2 kilograms per month (no more than half a kilogram per week) for those at the lower end of the scale, like Jennifer, with an upper limit of no more than 4 kilograms (1 kilogram per week) per month for those at the higher end, such as Max. If in doubt, 2 kilograms per month is a suitable goal.

Once your body accepts and becomes comfortable with your new weight after a month, you can work towards the next 2 kilogram weight loss the following month. However, don't be tempted to continue with weight loss during a weight maintenance month if you see weight coming off when you're on the scales. As ridiculous as it may sound, if this does occur and, for example, you notice a trend in weight loss between week 4 (month 1) and week 6 (month 1.5), you'll need to increase your energy intake by eating more over the following week or weeks: for example, weeks 6 (month 1.5) to 8 (month 2). This will ensure your weight returns to the start point (i.e. your weight at the start of the weight maintenance period).

Go on! Treat yourself!

This might mean allowing for more than one treat or takeaway/dining-out meal so that you stick as closely as possible to that 2 kilogram weight loss, or the specific weight-loss goal per month you set, or to ensure you keep your body weight steady during a weight maintenance month. Many patients I have helped see the weight coming off, get excited, and think they should ramp up their efforts so that more weight is lost. This is the complete opposite of what they should be doing, and I have to urge them to slow down and eat more to maintain their body weight. Thrilling as it may be to see weight rapidly coming off, you will not succeed if you do not follow this simple principle.

How do I get started?

First, go out and buy yourself a set of scales. It's a good idea to measure your body weight on the same set of scales each week. This is because there can be huge fluctuations between different scale types. The most helpful things to look for when purchasing scales include a large and clear display so you can easily read your body weight, and a weight-only default setting so that you don't have to scroll through the program control each time you weigh yourself. Always use your scales on a hard surface, as using them on carpet can return inaccurate and unreliable values.

If you don't want to invest in a set of scales, use the ones at your local sports club or gym, which are often pretty accurate. Stay clear of the scales that measure your body fat percentage, because these are generally poor quality and will only return meaningless results (body fat needs to be measured by gold standard techniques, such as dual-energy X-ray absorptiometry scans, which are costly and unnecessary unless you have a history of low bone mineral density).

How often should you weigh yourself?

I am often asked how often you should weigh yourself. Once a week is enough. Weigh yourself on the same day each week, in similar clothing, on the same scales and ideally at the same time of day. First thing before breakfast is a good time. There is no evidence to suggest that daily weighing is more effective than weekly for weight loss and weight maintenance. Yes, daily weighing can be effective but the problem is that some people who do it can become more focused on dieting and their body weight than on changing their lifestyle and behaviour. They also become alarmed by fluctuation in their weight, as people go up or down by as much as 1 to 2 kilograms in any given day, which is not a bad thing and to be expected.

It is therefore best just to monitor your weight each week rather than what is happening day to day – it is the trend over time that is the key thing to analyse.

Obsessing about your weight

Remember, the weight will come off naturally if you can focus on achieving a healthy lifestyle and following the steps in this book. If the scales have gone up – for example, 1.2 kilograms from Monday to Tuesday – this doesn't mean you have put on fat. It is just a fluctuation in body weight (most likely due to hydration), which needs to be ignored as it is completely normal. In short, please do not become obsessed by the number on the scales.

One of my clients, Felicity, began to become so focused on her weight that she started weighing herself three to four times a day. She became convinced that the fluctuations in her weight were real weight gain and consequently began to restrict her food intake, which eventually resulted in weight gain. I explained to Felicity that weighing herself so regularly was doing more harm than good and she decided, with my encouragement, to switch to a weekly weigh-in. Instead of restricting her food intake every time she looked at the scales, Felicity began to increase it, but from eating a range of wholesome, nutritious foods.

With this change, her mood improved, she felt better about herself, and her weight began to go down.

Note that if you start a resistance or weights training program (which I will touch on later) during a weight maintenance month, changes in body composition can happen very quickly, especially if you are mixing up your routine and sessions regularly, and hence your body weight is not relevant in this instance. If anything, your weight may be increasing if you are male or staying stable if you are female, but this is good, as you are setting yourself up for long-term success. Even for males, body weight will not increase if you are burning more energy than you are putting into your body. Remember, muscle weighs more than fat and is much more metabolically active, meaning that the more muscle to fat you have, the more energy you will be burning at rest.

How do you monitor your progress?

The most successful method is to record your weight on some form of tracker (electronic or paper) from week to week and monitor the trend over the given month. Some scales will also have wifi, which means you can check your measurements over a period of time with the accompanying smartphone application. I always provide my clients with blank templates they can use on their weight-loss journey, and that you can find at the back of this book. Visual is best – if you can plot your weight in an Excel spreadsheet, or something similar, you can see what is happening over time. If you are in the middle of a weight-loss period, the trend should be that it is going down roughly 1 to 2 kilograms over the month, and if it is a weight maintenance month it should even out across the month. An example of a recording chart for a weight-loss period is as follows (please note that each graph starts at a new week):

Body weight tracker for weight-loss month

Change in Body Weight over Time

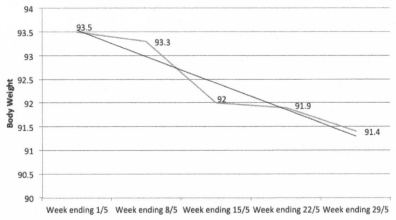

Note that the trend is that weight is going down over the course of the month (approximate 2 kilogram weight loss from a starting point of 93.5 kilograms to 91.4 kilograms). The black line is the linear trend.

Maintenance month

Think of your weight maintenance month as a reward month, because it often allows much more leniency regarding the 'treat' foods you can consume. Remember, you have to reset your body weight and convince your body that this is the new norm, before moving on to a weight-loss period again. Continue this and you can successfully lose 12 kilograms over a 12-month period as long as you follow the rest of the plan in this book. Any weight-loss goal can be set, but I highly recommend sticking to an upper limit of 12 kilograms over the course of the year.

Some people may only need to lose 2 to 5 kilograms, and they should adopt the same approach explained in this chapter to reprogram body weight. The key is to preserve your lean muscle mass – and some physical activity will play a key role in this (more on this later). You will then be setting yourself up for much easier long-term weight maintenance.

I always tell my patients that if you can keep the weight off for five years, it is like being in remission with a lower chance of recurrence – in this case, of weight regain. Two examples of weight maintenance periods are as follows:

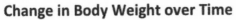

(A) Body weight tracker for weight maintenance month

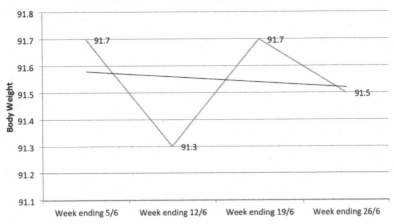

In this example, note that the trend evens out over the course of the month to maintain the 2 kilogram weight loss from the previous month. The black line is the linear trend.

(B) Body weight tracker for weight maintenance month

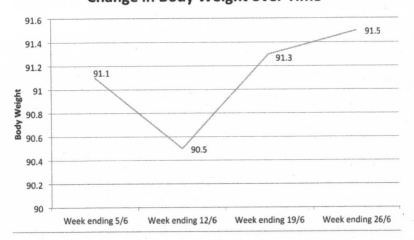

Note that in this instance, there is a trend towards weight loss over the first two weeks (from 91.4 kilograms at the end of the weight-loss period in the weight-loss graph to 90.5 kilograms in the week ending 12/6) in what should be a weight maintenance period. As a result, the person has corrected this by allowing for a higher energy intake to ensure their body weight corrects back to the starting point of the weight maintenance month (which was 91.4 kilograms – see the weight loss graph).

Body weight tracker for a 12-month period

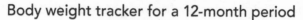

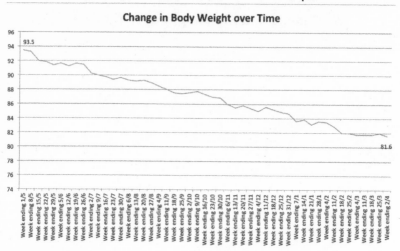

In this 12-month chart, the weight is decreasing by approximately 2 kilograms each month and then maintained for the following month, equating approximately to a 12 kilogram weight loss over the year. Body weight is 93.5 kilograms at the baseline and 81.6 kilograms after approximately 12 months.

The long-term effect

During my time consulting with patients in both the private and public sectors, I have had huge success with this Interval Weight Loss plan. New leading research[5] supports this approach, and the way it allows people to test small changes to their lifestyle and the effect they have on their body weight.

The proof, of course, is also in the pudding. It is quite common for me many years down the track to run into people I have helped on their weight-loss journey. At my local swimming pool, I now frequently bump into a lady I helped at the beginning of my career. Every time I see her she says, 'Look at me, Nick! It's been all these years and I've kept the weight off!' I can honestly say it makes my day.

CHAPTER 3

WHAT TO EAT

'You don't need a silver fork to eat
good food.' – *Paul Prudhomme*

So, now we've discussed how to monitor your weight loss and trick your body into believing it's at its new set point, but how do we lose those 1–2 kilos every other month?

What I am going to tell you in this chapter is not to follow a set diet plan, like the majority of weight-loss books do, but instead to eat as much as you can – but of the *right types of foods*. There is no calorie counting involved. The most successful weight-loss maintenance stories I have researched are those where people have eaten a large volume of food and participated in, and enjoyed, a wide variety of physical activities. Think back to Felicity in the previous chapter, who began weighing herself obsessively.

Her greatest success came when she stopped restricting her food intake.

Yes, you can eat as much food as you like, providing you stick to wholesome, filling, low-energy foods that are high in nutrition the majority of the time – more on this later. This means staying clear of processed food coming out of a packet, or food made from ingredients coming out of a packet. Such processed foods are often very low in fibre and high in sugar and fat, and hence do not fill us up the same way as do foods from their natural source.

One of my clients, Jacob, was struggling to lose weight despite telling me he ate a 'healthy' diet and that he wasn't overeating. When I asked him to keep a food diary, however, it turned out that the vast majority of his food intake was from processed foods. He was delighted to find that when he switched to fresh food he was not only eating more but also losing weight. He also said he had more energy, which is so often the case when you start to eat properly.

Remember, we want to do all we can to increase our metabolism or prevent it from slowing down, which occurs when you restrict your food intake. We also want to prevent an increase in appetite hormones associated with energy restriction, telling us to eat, which results in weight regain. So, eat before the hunger pangs set in. Focus on eating more at the start of the day and eat small, frequent meals, to prevent a situation where you overeat at the next main meal (see the meal plans in Part 2 of this book).

Five meals a day

I believe that five meals a day should form the basis of your meal plan, rather than the standard three. The majority of your food intake should be in the first half of the day, so that your appetite will not be as great in the afternoon or evening. As American author and nutritionist Adelle Davis said, 'Eat breakfast like a king, lunch like a prince, and dinner like a pauper.' Breakfast should be your biggest meal and dinner your smallest. This means you will now need to eat dinner off small crockery, such as a bread and butter plate, or from a rice bowl.

Whenever you are hungry, you should eat. And each day your food intake should be based on the following:

1. Unlimited fruit and vegetables (all are suitable but enjoy a variety).

2. Plenty (minimum 2–3 serves) of skim or low-fat dairy (milk and yoghurt, preferably skim/no fat or low fat options, but watch out for no fat/low fat yoghurt that is higher in added sugar). Keep your cheese intake to

a maximum of once per week, which still allows you to enjoy a little!

3. Handful of nuts (preferably walnuts or almonds) and seeds (approximately 30g or 12 nuts).

4. Inclusion of a 'wholegrain' carbohydrate with three meals per day (for example, wholegrain bread). Wholegrain foods contain all components of the original grain seed (i.e. the bran, germ and endosperm). All of these must be present for food to qualify as wholegrain.

5. Inclusion of lean or 'heart smart' cuts of meat (trim all visible forms of fat off the meat), or fish of any type. Plenty of fish (tinned tuna or salmon is an easy and convenient option for increasing your fish intake), and have legumes of any type, or eggs, each day. You should select one of these to accompany each of the three main meals.

6. Treats such as ice-cream and chocolate no more than once a week.

7. Fast food or dining out no more than once a week.

Gluten intolerance

For those with *diagnosed* gluten intolerance, and I emphasise 'diagnosed' (i.e. those with coeliac disease), or with lactose intolerance, this plan still applies to you – it applies to everyone. Simply include alternatives to wheat products, such as buckwheat, corn, quinoa or rice, and lactose-free dairy products in your diet. If you suspect you may have gluten sensitivity but have not been diagnosed with coeliac disease, I would recommend following a gluten-free diet purely for improved well-being, as nutritional consequences associated with coeliac disease and malnutrition will not be relevant to you and will not help you lose weight.

Emergency food

For those days when you are genuinely time-poor or don't get home from work till very late, it's okay to have some frozen meals in the freezer, such as Healthy Choice, Lean Cuisine or Weight Watchers. These are suitable for emergencies and are portion-controlled, nutritionally balanced meals (giving you adequate carbohydrate, protein and fat). However, I stress that they should only be for emergencies and not form the bulk of your meal plan.

You might find that you are eating more with this new way of life – this is not only allowed but encouraged. As mentioned before, I don't want you to count calories. I just want you to eat regularly and to eat to your appetite (which we will touch on in a later chapter). In most cases, people do find themselves eating much more than they used to, but with a focus on a variety of low-energy, nutrient-rich, filling foods. Often you will find your caloric intake still lessens and even if it hasn't, you are preserving or increasing your metabolic rate and setting yourself up for long-term success.

Food myths

Some nutrition myths die but others live on forever. Nowadays we are presented with so much conflicting information that it's hard to know what we should and shouldn't eat. Gossip magazines, current affairs programs that promote fad diets, not to mention the internet, only add to this confusion. Unless you are reading academic peer-reviewed literature, diets must all be ignored, and even then, you need to be able to critique the literature based on the study design, number of subjects involved, journal ranking, or impact factor in its field. Open-access journals make things even more confusing. Sifting through them is an art in itself but, unless you are really keen, you can now ignore them all as I am providing you with knowledge based on proven science. The following will dispel some of the myths surrounding food.

Oil

Many people are wary of oil, but they shouldn't be if it is used correctly. What sort of oil should you use? Olive oil or canola oil only. Both oils are low in saturated fat and high in monounsaturated fat compared with all other oils (this is good!). Canola oil is a cheaper alternative to olive oil. With respect to the range of olive oils, it doesn't matter if you are buying 'extra virgin', 'virgin', or 'pure'. However, if you can afford it, buy 'extra virgin' olive oil. It has a distinct flavour and is darker in colour when compared with 'pure' or regular olive oil, as it has not been refined, making it a suitable option for salad dressings. When you're cooking, the same also applies – use olive or canola oil only; just don't let the oil smoke, as this means it has gone beyond its smoking point and is now rancid. If this happens, you have the temperature too high and you need to start again. Unless you are deep frying (which you shouldn't be anyway), olive or canola oil have suitable smoking points for all types of cooking, including stir-fries. Due to the slightly lower smoke point of extra virgin olive oil, pure or regular olive oil can be a more suitable option for cooking. Spray bottles also allow for better portion control when cooking.

Nuts

Nuts are often considered fattening but there is no evidence to support this. What sort of nuts should you eat? Walnuts and almonds provide the best nutrient profile. Buy them in their raw, natural or dry-roasted form. If you are looking for an alternative to these two types of nuts, you can enjoy all others occasionally but be sure to buy unsalted and raw, or dry-roasted.

Vegetables

Are there vegetables to avoid? No. You can eat all vegetables, and starchy vegetables such as potatoes will not make you fat, unless you are having them deep-fried in oil all the time. Include a mixture of all types and colours and buy according to season. Frozen is just as good as fresh, as frozen vegetables are snap-frozen at the time of picking and their nutrients retained.

Fruit

Are there fruits to avoid? No. Again, as with vegetables, you can enjoy all types of fruit. They are high in water and packed full of nutrients.

Dairy

Will dairy food make you fat? Absolutely not! As with nuts, there is no evidence to suggest that dairy causes weight gain. However, stick to yoghurt and milk the majority of the time, and have cheese only once a week. This is because even low-fat cheese is still very high in fat, particularly saturated fat, which can increase your cholesterol level, and while this doesn't cause weight gain it does block arteries which leads to heart attacks. Low-fat milk and yoghurt is better than full fat because low fat has the same amount of nutrition (for example, protein, calcium) with lower energy content, notably from saturated fat. Even better is skim or no fat milk or yoghurt, which again contains the same nutrition as full fat without the wasted energy intake. They are acquired tastes, so trial low fat first, and a mixture of brands to find what you like best, and then, if you can, trial skim or no fat next. You will get used to them, trust me! There is no need for alternatives to dairy, such as soy or almond products, however many people include them for taste which is also fine.

Eggs

How many eggs should you eat? You don't need to limit eggs. They are high in protein, containing all nine essential amino acids, and are very nutritious. Despite the misconception that eggs should be avoided due to their cholesterol and fat content, they are not bad for you, and if anything they raise your good cholesterol, which protects you from cardiovascular disease. Most recently, the American Dietary Guidelines were changed to abolish the limit on cholesterol intake per day (previously no more than 300 mg a day), which further supports the inclusion of eggs in the diet. However, this doesn't mean you can include them as part of a staple 'egg and bacon diet'. They should be eaten boiled or poached, and if fried they should be cooked in a small amount of olive oil spray.

Carbs

Do you need to restrict your carbohydrate intake? No, as I've said, carbs do not make you fat, unless you are including a lot of processed, refined carbohydrate foods, such as white bread, pastries, bakery goods, pre-packaged foods like muesli bars, biscuits, muffins, pancakes, noodles, bagels, pretzels and corn chips. Anything that is not processed is okay. High-glycaemic foods – meaning they raise our blood sugar level rapidly – such as potato, are fine although it's also good to include low-glycaemic alternatives such as sweet potato because they do not raise our blood sugar level as fast and therefore provide sustained energy over a longer period of time. And eating carbs at night is also fine. It doesn't matter what time of the day you are eating carbs, what matters is the type of food you are eating and how many calories you are putting into your mouth over the course of the day. Food intake is only bad at night if you are comfort eating. There is no evidence that restricting carbs after 2pm or not eating carbs at night help with weight loss.

The South Beach diet, which was written by a cardiologist and included some principles of a healthy diet, has led people to think that carbs are to be avoided at all costs. The same can be said of the Atkins diet. There is a component at the start of the program whereby carbs are stripped from or reduced in the diet and, as a result, you appear to have instant success. People see rapid weight loss on the scales and develop the notion that it must be carbohydrates that cause all the weight gain. Well, this is not true. If you are eating the correct type of carbohydrates (wholegrain or low glycaemic index ones), you are including many of the nutrients that are vital for a balanced diet. Stripping carbohydrates from the diet will achieve more success in the short term, due to the water carrying capacity of carbohydrates (i.e. you strip carbohydrates and you strip water from the body) and various other factors, such as the energy process in breaking down protein, but a low-carbohydrate diet will have no greater success in the long term.

It is scientifically proven[6] that high carbohydrate versus low carbohydrate diets achieve the same amount of weight loss over 12 months or longer. So, don't think carbohydrates are the culprit – they certainly aren't, as long as you are not eating a highly processed and refined diet. There are other similar diets based on the same principles that have an even more restrictive initial intensive phase of low carb intake, such as the Dr Atkins New Diet Revolution and, as I've mentioned, the Palaeo diet. These type of diets are also often lacking in other essential nutrients such as fibre, which is important for gut health, and calcium, which is important for bone health, and so they should be avoided.

Coffee

Do I need to cut out coffee? No, absolutely not. Coffee is one way to increase your dairy consumption. A skim milk-based coffee (or full fat, if you must) provides a serve of dairy and a snack option for morning or afternoon tea. Try to stick to no more than two cups per day, due to the stimulant effect of caffeine. There is no link between coffee consumption and increased risk of cancer or cardiovascular disease, and coffee consumption has in fact been associated with many health benefits[7]. However, coffee brewing methods that don't use a filter, common in countries such as Turkey, may increase your blood fat levels and should be avoided.

Coffee versus tea

Is coffee better than tea? No. Both coffee and tea contain antioxidants, which mop up free radicals – known to be harmful substances in our bodies that cause cancer. Both tea and coffee contain caffeine, unless you are having herbal tea.

Chocolate

Is chocolate good for me? Yes, dark chocolate is full of antioxidants but it is also high in energy and saturated fat, so must be kept as a treat and eaten only once a week. Milk chocolate or white chocolate should be kept to a minimum, as such forms of chocolate have been through greater processing, meaning that they contain less of the original cocoa bean and are much lower in nutritive value than dark chocolate.

Artificial sweeteners

Do artificial sweeteners cause cancer? No, the evidence does not show this, despite what you might have read or been told. More importantly, artificial sweeteners can play an important role in the diet, as they displace added sugars commonly associated with some foods and beverages. Again, despite what you may have been told or read, they do not increase appetite. Nevertheless, it's better to go without any kind of sweetener – artificial or otherwise – if you can.

Malabsorption

Is it possible that being unable to process certain foods, such as wheat, will make you fat? No, absolutely not. If you can't absorb a particular food, you are likely to get side effects and experience malabsorption, which will more likely result in malnutrition and weight loss. So, if you are avoiding gluten because you think it makes you fat, this is nonsense, and sadly there are a lot of people making money out of this claim. An endoscopy (gold standard test) or blood test is used to diagnose coeliac disease, and those who are diagnosed need to follow a gluten-free diet. Sufferers of gluten intolerance will experience side effects such as diarrhoea, bloating, reflux and malabsorption of their food due to flattening of the microvilli in the small intestine.

Butter and margarine

Butter or margarine? Neither. Margarines that are marketed to lower our bad (low-density lipoprotein) cholesterol levels need to be consumed in large volumes to have an effect. These are the margarines that you see on television commercials that claim to reduce cholesterol. For example, you need to have 25 grams of a plant sterol margarine spread per day (which equals 5 slices of bread, with 5 grams – or a teaspoon – on every slice) to have a cholesterol-lowering effect. You are better off switching to avocado or olive oil as your spread of choice.

Supplements

Many people ask me what supplements they should use. In the majority of cases, most of the benefits of vitamins and minerals come from eating food rich in that nutrient, rather than supplements themselves. A well-balanced diet will avoid the need for vitamin and nutrient supplements. In fact, if you are eating a varied diet, as proposed in this book, you will receive little to no benefit from a multi-vitamin supplement. Often you will just be excreting the vitamins through your urine. For example, an excess of vitamin B2 (riboflavin) will be indicated by urine being a dark fluorescent colour.

However, there are some situations where supplements may be beneficial, such as when you have to avoid certain food. And, of course, folic acid and iodine are essential for women trying to fall pregnant and during pregnancy. It is beyond the scope and purpose of this book to review all supplements that are currently on the market – there are thousands of them. However, the only ones that I believe you may need to take are the following:

Omega 3: There are health benefits associated with omega 3 consumption, specifically relating to a reduction in inflammatory markers and blood fats in the body. However, the best way to get these benefits is to eat foods rich in omega 3, such as fish, as supplements may not have the same effect. If you don't eat fish, you should take a fish oil capsule every day. Stick to the odourless supplement if you prefer and an intake of 3000 mg per day.

Calcium: If you avoid dairy or are not getting enough calcium-rich foods other than dairy (for example, tinned fish with bones, tofu and almonds) in your diet, you should include a calcium supplement every day. Calcium is important for bone health and preventing osteoporosis, also known as brittle bones. Dairy foods are the richest sources of calcium and are of the highest bioavailability, meaning there is a higher absorption rate of calcium from them.

Vitamin D: In conjunction with calcium, vitamin D is also important for bone health and preventing osteoporosis. Natural sunlight is the richest source of vitamin D and we only require very small amounts each day. A 5–10 minute walk outside will be enough to meet daily requirements.

Vitamin D is also found in some food sources, such as eggs. However, for those who see little to no sunlight each week, a vitamin D supplement will most likely be needed. Please consult with your general practitioner if you are concerned or have not had your vitamin D levels tested. There is a simple blood test you can have to establish whether you are at risk of osteoporosis.

Glucosamine: There is some clinical evidence to support its use as a way of improving joint health. For those with a history of, for example, knee or hip pain, benefits may be gained from a supplement of glucosamine at an intake of 2000 mg per day.

Iron: For those who have childbearing potential and a low dietary intake of iron from animal sources, an iron supplement may be needed. Red meat is the richest source of bio-available iron and should be included in the food plan two times weekly. Symptoms of low iron include tiredness and lack of energy. A deficiency can be detected through an iron studies blood test.

Vitamin B12: A vitamin B12 supplement is required for those who are vegan and avoid all animal products, or those who are deficient in intrinsic factor (an enzyme required to bind vitamin B12 in the stomach). Those at risk of this deficiency include people who are over 70 years of age. A deficiency can be detected by a blood test and it is treated by a vitamin B12 subcutaneous injection. This can be provided by a general practitioner or a nurse.

How much is too much?

Let me reiterate: you can eat as much as you like each day, but what you eat must be based on the core food groups mentioned earlier. It doesn't matter how much you put on your plate or how frequently you eat. The only restriction is that you must follow the 'tunnel plan' – i.e. from big to small throughout the day, so that your evening meal must fit on a bread and butter plate or in a rice bowl. Eat as much as you like at breakfast; lunch then needs to be a little smaller than breakfast; and dinner the smallest of all. Again, my suggestion is to eat big at breakfast, and if that means having something before you leave for work and then again when you arrive at work (a two-part breakfast), then that is fine! Remember to include small meals, such as fruit and nuts, in between main meals to help prevent hunger setting in.

Recognising when you're hungry

A key focus of this plan is to eat as much as you can — to eat plenty of food, to eat to your appetite, and to base the bulk of your intake on the core food groups that I have mentioned. Most of the time when you think you are hungry, you more than likely are. In this instance, your hunger cues will be telling you when you really need to eat. For most people, it's okay just to eat when their brain is telling them that they are hungry. However, some people who have dieted for years become unable to listen to their body, and so don't know how to eat normally or recognise when they're really hungry. In this instance, it is best to eat small, regular meals to prevent periods of over-eating due to excessive hunger.

Temptation at work

For those who have jobs where they are regularly bored and graze on food to pass the time, or, conversely, find themselves so stressed that they comfort eat, the work environment can cause issues. In either case, you need to get up and move as often as possible to avoid the temptation to eat. And factor in, as well, the number of times you unthinkingly eat a slice of cake for morning or afternoon tea because a colleague is leaving, or having a birthday, or going on maternity leave, or the company's just landed a big contract ... It adds up!

After dinner

After dinner is the main time you need to be wary of, as the end of the day is often a time of relaxation. We tend to associate relaxation with eating, especially when taking part in activities such as watching television, and often snack without thinking about what we are putting in our mouths. What should you do when this happens? First of all, think about what your body is telling you – are you really hungry? You not long ago had dinner, so perhaps all you need is a warm drink such as a herbal tea, or to distract yourself by doing something productive (for example, sewing, knitting, reading a book, playing with the kids, de-cluttering your cupboards or creating a 'to do' list – more on this later).

I love this time of the day because it is when you can get the most rewards. If you can distract yourself with a productive activity, you will feel a huge sense of achievement and prevent yourself from eating something that you more than likely didn't need. Remember, you are probably only reaching for a snack because of the association of food with relaxation. You will quickly forget that you were even thinking about food if you distract yourself, and before you know it you will be getting into bed. So, why not start a new project or hobby? Anything to keep your mind busy. It doesn't matter what it is; if it's enjoyable and constructive, it's worthwhile.

Keeping a journal

One way of distracting yourself in the evening is to keep a journal. Some of the people I have helped most success-fully over the years have attributed a large amount of their success to keeping a journal of their day-to-day lives (this is, at least, a way to kick start their success). This is espe-cially important at the start of your journey to the new you, as it allows you to reflect on certain behaviours that may be acting as barriers and hindrances in your life. This journal is for recording your thoughts rather than just recording what you eat, although you can do that too if you think it will help you. It means keeping a log of things you do in your day – what you did, the time you did it, how you felt, your energy level, what you enjoyed, what you didn't enjoy, and maybe what you think you could work on.

If you prefer not to write, it can just be a journal of pictures that reflect your thoughts. At the end of each week, when you record your weight on your weekly tracker, reflect back on your journal and see how it matches up to your progress.

Again, like everything else, your journal can be on paper or kept electronically. If you don't want to do it in the evening, you can do it on public transport when you go to work or any other time that suits you. You don't have to record every activity you have done. It could just be a reflection of what you did and didn't enjoy in your day.

The process of writing everything down will help make you feel good – you can re-live the day's events without any fear or stress.

Remember, the benefit of a journal is that no one else sees it – just you! You are the only one to reflect on it. It might be your food choices you are monitoring, how many negative thoughts you have, how often you report being happy, how energetic you feel. It doesn't matter what it is, as long as you are reporting it. If there are things in there that are constantly popping up and that are making you unhappy, you need to do something about them and make appropriate changes – because these things might be big enough to stop you from breaking through and succeeding. Similarly, make note of the things that regularly result in happiness, as you need to keep repeating them. Your journal serves, in a way, to build healthy habits; and, importantly, forces you to become aware of your actions and behaviours and the reasons behind them.

Evening exercise

Another way to distract yourself in the evening is to exercise. Whether it's a stroll around the neighbourhood, a run on the treadmill, or a ride on a stationary bike, these are very constructive activities. You may even have the luxury of being able to do the latter in front of the television. You see, it's okay to associate television viewing with exercise, because now every time you sit down in front of the television, you will be thinking about exercise and not food!

Skipping meals

For those who lead an especially busy and hectic life, comfort eating is much less of an issue, if at all, during the day. In fact, the opposite applies for those who are busy – they forget, or don't make time, to eat. However, this is one of the worst things you can do. By skipping meals, all you are doing is setting yourself up for failure. In this instance, you must set reminders – on your computer or phone – to eat and force yourself to take a break for five minutes to do so. If you can eat something healthy every two to three hours, you will prevent yourself from overeating and making poor food choices at main mealtimes. More importantly, you will prevent that ever-so-common situation where you come home from work and are ravenous because you haven't eaten all day, and reach for anything you can get your hands on.

Drinking enough

Are you drinking enough? No, not alcohol! I mean water. Water plays a vital role in a healthy lifestyle. Not only does it ensure you remain hydrated so that your cells can function properly, it plays an important part in delaying the ageing process by keeping your skin healthy. Basically, dehydration means your body functioning declines. You should be drinking a total of 2 litres of non-caffeinated beverages every day – the bulk of this will come from water, and perhaps skim/low-fat milk. Stay clear of fruit juices because they are a concentrated form of energy (even if they are 100 per cent natural juice with no added sugar) and you get much more satiety from eating a piece of fruit as opposed to having a glass of juice.

The key is to take a water bottle everywhere you go, and to focus the majority of your fluid intake during the first half of the day, slowing down after 4pm to ensure it doesn't affect your sleeping routine. If you drink too much later in the day, you might find that you are getting up frequently during the night to urinate. Really, you shouldn't be getting up more than once a night to do this, to avoid compromising sleep quality. If a water bottle is a nuisance and you don't like to carry one around, then ensure you have one on your work desk and fill it up at the start of every day. If you are never at your desk, have two glasses of water before every meal, apart from the evening meal. This also serves as a good mindfulness eating technique. Next time you think you may be hungry but you're not entirely sure, have a couple of glasses of water, wait a couple of minutes, and if you still have hunger cues – eat!

If you are drinking 2 litres of fluid per day, you will be hydrated and your urine should appear relatively clear. For those who still aren't sure whether they're properly hydrated, there are self-assessment scales to help (i.e. the classical 8-point urine colour scale[8]). Anything in the safe zone (1–3) means you are well hydrated, and anything in the danger zone (4–8) means you are dehydrated. If you get to the stage where you are thirsty, you are already dehydrated. Drinking water can be seasonally driven (i.e. based on temperature), so during the colder winter months I would suggest focusing on warmer decaffeinated beverages to keep your fluid intake up, such as herbal infused teas (chamomile, lemon and ginger and peppermint). You can also occasionally include sparkling water (mineral or soda water) as an alternative. This is a great suggestion for when you are eating out because it creates the feeling that you are treating yourself to more than just regular tap water. While the salt content in such beverages is low, it is still important that they do not comprise the majority of your fluid intake.

Alcohol

Alcohol can be enjoyed in moderation and a low level of intake can increase your good (high-density lipoprotein) cholesterol level in the blood, meaning it reduces plaque accumulation in your arteries. High levels will cause the opposite to happen. You should have no more than 2 standard drinks (both males and females) and include 2 alcohol-free days a week.[9]

How much is a standard drink?
Can/stubbie low-strength beer = 0.8 standard drink
Can/stubbie mid-strength beer = 1 standard drink
Can/stubbie full-strength beer = 1.4 standard drinks
100ml wine (13.5% alcohol) = 1 standard drink
30ml nip spirits = 1 standard drink
Can spirits (approx 5–7% alcohol) = 1.2 to 2.4
    standard drinks

Being present in the moment

Mindful eating is all about being present in the current moment – eating with intention, and paying attention to what you are doing. You need to disassociate eating from other activities. The next time a computer or phone reminder goes off to tell you that you are due a break, walk away from the screen or desk, and eat in an area that is not associated with work or pleasure, away from technological distractions. It should only take you about five minutes to do so (you may need to go to the fridge anyway, to grab one of your snacks) and if you sit for most of the day at work, this is a golden opportunity to move. Importantly, food should be enjoyed, so eat slowly and ensure you appreciate what you are eating.

The evening meal routine

It's important to start implementing an evening meal routine. This meal should always be eaten at the dining table to prevent the association of television with food. We are programmed to certain behaviours. If you always eat your dinner in front of the television, you are more likely to associate the television with food at any other given time. Quite apart from that, it is the perfect time to either sit by yourself or to have dinner with your partner or family and reflect on your day. Eating at the dinner table slows down the eating process so that you focus on chewing your food properly, appreciating and enjoying the meal. You will also find that you eat a lot slower when you are sitting at the dinner table, as opposed to sitting on the couch in front of the television.

My grandfather used to always tell me that the slowest one wins the race. He never had a weight problem and he had a huge appetite and enjoyed all types of food, including the occasional sweet, but he would always be the last person to finish eating. It may seem ridiculous, but next time you are at the dinner table, time how long it takes you to eat your meal and then write it down. Slow down your meal each time, until you get to a point where you realise that you are actually chewing and enjoying your food. You will often find that it is double the amount of time that you were taking to eat your evening meal at the beginning, or that it's now taking the same amount of time to eat half the amount of the evening meal you were having before because you have started eating off a bread and butter plate, or out of a rice-sized bowl.

CHAPTER 4

EATING OUT

'Shame is a soul-eating emotion.'
– *Carl Gustav Jung*

The golden rule of dining out or getting takeaway food is to only do it once a week. If you are concerned about what to eat when you go out, you have the wrong mentality. Success comes with liberation. On the day of the week when you go out, you can eat whatever you like, so you don't need to be worried about what you are selecting off the menu. Sure, the really health conscious will stick to healthier options but that is their preference. If you like the look of the laksa on the menu, then get the laksa!

The same applies to what I consider 'treat' foods – have them just once a week and have anything you want. Maybe it's something from the local ice-cream shop or a slice of cake you love – it doesn't matter what it is, as long as it's only once a week. And, as I've said previously, you may be able to have more 'treat' foods during your weight maintenance months, to ensure your weight does not drop. The key to success is to enjoy everything and not to exclude certain foods that you enjoy. If you do exclude those foods, you are still adopting the 'diet' mentality, and you need to go back to Chapter 1 and start reading all over again.

If you are regularly eating out more than once a week, lunch and dinners included, then you need to take a step back and think for a second – why are you eating out more than once a week? Is it a social thing? If so, re-shape your social life so that, for example, you meet a friend for a walk rather than for food and drinks. Is it because you need to work more on your organisational skills and planning? If so, read the next chapter, on getting organised. Once you have mastered this, you will be well on the way to your new healthy lifestyle.

Special occasions

If you are at a birthday celebration, some other kind of special occasion, or out with friends, you can eat anything you like if it's your treat meal. If it's not, however, think carefully about your food selection. Despite what some people might think, foods such as banana bread are not healthy because they have banana as an ingredient. Think of these foods as equivalent to having a slice of cake.

Business lunches

If you lead a corporate life, constantly going to lunch meetings and evening functions, you are in a difficult situation. If they are really unavoidable (and this is sometimes not the case), you need to be selective about your menu choices and stick with entrée-sized meals, as opposed to main-course sizes. When we eat out, we tend to consume double the energy content of a home-cooked meal. Why is this? Because the chef is doing all they can to get you to come back to their restaurant. This often means upping flavours with liberal amounts of energy-dense foods such as oil, cream and butter (to name a few), and lots of salt. So, if you really can't lessen the number of times you eat out, then you need to be selective in your restaurant choice and selective in your menu choices.

I would suggest staying clear of hot food, and trying to stick to cold food options, like sushi and cafés where you can control what goes in your sandwich. For those instances where you are not able to select the dining venue, here are a few suggestions of cuisines. The general rule, though, is to control portion size and to avoid fried dishes.

American
Choose salad-based meals but ask for the dressing on the side.

Australian pub food

Opt for salmon or steak but, instead of hot chips, ask for salad with dressing on the side, or steamed/boiled vegetables with no added condiments (such as butter).

Chinese

Choose vegetable- or fish-based dishes, avoid fried dishes, and share plates with others if possible. Ask for boiled rice instead of fried.

Fast-food road stops

Select pre-made sandwiches or salads. Even though they will contain added condiments that you would not use at home, this is a much healthier and more nutritious option than burgers, fries or fried chicken.

French

Select dishes such as steamed mussels or grilled fish, and salads with vinaigrette dressing.

Greek

Opt for grilled meats and vegetables, fish cooked in tomatoes (plaki), or Greek salad.

Indian

Choose steamed rice and tomato-based dishes. Avoid curries made with coconut milk or cream.

Italian
Select pastas with tomato-based sauces (entrée size) or salads. Avoid energy-dense appetisers such as garlic bread.

Japanese
Select sushi or sashimi, miso soup, edamame, or seaweed salad. Avoid fried foods.

Korean
Try different varieties of kimchi and bibimbap, and avoid fried foods. (Korea has one of the lowest rates of over-weight and obese people, so this may be a cuisine to have more often.)

Malaysian
Share plates with others if possible. Opt for salads and steamed rice instead of fried. Avoid dishes that are largely noodle or rice based.

Mediterranean
Salads, fish or meat-based dishes (with tomato-based sauces).

Mexican
Select grilled fish or meat, salsa, jalapeños, chicken or beef fajitas or enchiladas (specify no cheese and no sour cream).

Thai
Choose a stir-fried dish with vegetables, or try chilli beef (neua pad prik), and share plates with others if possible.

Avoid fried spring rolls and try fresh spring rolls. Opt for steamed rice instead of fried.

Vietnamese

Opt for rice paper rolls, salads, steamed whole fish, or traditional soups such as pho.

Travel

Travel is often thought of as another challenging time in life, especially if we find ourselves on the road all the time because of work. The best option when you travel interstate or abroad is to book an apartment, rather than a hotel, so you can prepare and cook your own food. You may have a lot more time on your hands when you travel (for example, with no family around), so use it to exercise and explore the sights. If you do find yourself in a hotel, or on a trip or all-inclusive holiday that has an endless supply of buffet meals, you'll need to be careful with your choices and restrict the volume of food you are eating. As suggested earlier for your evening meals, it's a good idea to use a bread and butter sized plate, rather than loading up a dinner sized plate, for all meals. Travel is a time to capitalise on, and often a time for weight loss, rather than weight gain, due to the extra exercise you might be doing. It's a time in your life where you can create an opportunity, so don't fear it but, rather, be excited by it!

Café-style eating

As I've touched on, café-style eating is a more suitable option than the high-energy hot lunch you might otherwise have had (especially in business situations where you are meeting with a client). It allows for the opportunity to control what you are putting in your body. This is even more relevant when you are in a familiar area and know what eateries are on offer. Once you have established a repertoire of places where you can vouch for the meal and service quality, you will have greater control over the food you will be eating. You want a place where you know that there are no hidden extras (for example, butter, margarine, salt and other condiments) and that you will walk away from feeling good after having a meal there. Avoid pre-packaged or pre-prepared meals, where you cannot be certain of their exact composition. If you want a spread on your bread, avoid butter or margarine and ask for avocado. Ensure your carbohydrate source is a wholegrain option, and your protein source is not fried or pre-prepared in an abundance of high-energy condiments like full-fat mayonnaise.

Most importantly, next time you go out, reflect on whether it was an enjoyable experience. If it wasn't, then don't go back there. Build a portfolio of places that imprint a positive experience on your mind, with a sense of control over what you are eating. After all, the eating experience must be enjoyable as well as healthy.

CHAPTER 5

GETTING ORGANISED

'If you fail to plan, you are planning to fail.' – Benjamin Franklin

The wide variety of food you'll be eating may mean a few different trips to different distributors, if you have time. For example, to the fruit market, the butcher, the fish market and the supermarket. If time doesn't allow for this, you may just be taking the one trip to the supermarket. However, if your budget is of concern, as it is for most of us, the main way to save is to buy direct from the wholesalers (for example, fruit markets, and large bulk-buy suppliers such as Costco or low-cost supermarkets like Aldi if you have either of them near you).

Whichever way you approach it, the food for the week must be purchased at the same time. This will save you time throughout the week as those impulse buys on a daily basis will only lead to extra centimetres around the waist and money poorly spent. The fewer times you go to the supermarket, the better, as I consider this another huge danger zone. We are spoilt for choice in the supermarkets, and they are strategically organised by the multinational companies so that energy-dense, nutrient-poor foods surround us everywhere – even at the check-outs as we wait in line to pay for our groceries.

Alex, a young male who I helped for many years, used to always lose his self-control in the supermarket. It took a while for him to confess that this was his biggest weakness. We set a goal for Alex only to grocery shop immediately after eating. This ensured he was not hungry and tempted to buy foods that were not on his shopping list. He found that a good time was on weekends, just after breakfast (of course, the biggest meal of the day). He also found that there were two to three aisles that could be skipped altogether – those that contained soft drinks, chips and confectionery, which were a huge temptation for him.

Home delivery

If you have the money to do so and live in a city, you can have everything home delivered with very little effort required. The foods you regularly purchase are saved in your account, so that you don't miss things. This then avoids the pain of having to go to the supermarket for any missed items. Online food shopping and delivery are particularly helpful for not only managing your grocery list but also saving you money, as the relevant supermarket chain will alert you to when certain foods are on sale.

If you enjoy the food-shopping experience, which many of us do, and prefer to select your own fruit and vegetables, keep a list of foods you need, to keep you on track. You will also need to shop immediately after eating so that you are not hungry and tempted to buy food that is not on your list. A good time is after breakfast, as Alex found.

The majority of your list will by the same every week, especially if you have specific meals on different days. This can be logged electronically on a smartphone, using some great applications such as Wunderlist and AnyList, to name a couple.

List of meals

Next, sit down and make a list of meals that you, your partner and your family really like. Recipe manager Paprika is a user-friendly smartphone application that allows you to find recipes you like on the web, and add all the items you need to a grocery list and remove the ones you already have. On the whole, all you need are six or seven different meals for the week (see Part 2 of this book for inspiration). That is enough variety for you to repeat them week in, week out, especially if you, your partner, or your family enjoy them. That way, your shopping list remains consistent and the stress is taken out of food shopping.

As I mentioned, the cheapest way to save money on grocery shopping is to actually break up the experience into two to four different trips to wholesalers, providing you have suppliers close by your home or workplace. For example, go to the fruit and vegetable market and get whatever you can according to the budget you have. You can never have too much fruit and vegetables, as they will form the basis of each of your meals.

Then go to the wholesale meat distributor/local butcher or fish market, and again purchase whatever you can with the budget you have. If money is tight, just buy enough red meat for two meals over the week and use tinned fish to supplement lunch or evening meals, as it is cheaper. Remember, you can freeze the meat if it's less expensive to buy larger amounts. And lastly, a visit to one of your wholesale or retail suppliers to purchase the remaining items (for example, dairy, eggs, legumes, lentils, nuts, seeds, wholegrain bread). Steer clear of processed foods out of a packet (for example, biscuits, chips, muesli bars) because the majority of the foods you need to eat should be in their raw, whole or unprocessed form. However, tinned foods such as fish, tomatoes, legumes and lentils, to name a few, are fantastic, cheap, healthy staples that you should always have in stock.

Good habits

As I mentioned earlier, we live in an environment that makes it challenging to lose and maintain weight. We are surrounded by fast food outlets and convenience foods and, as a consequence, we are putting far more high-energy, nutrient-poor food into our bodies, often due to poor planning. Modern technology also encourages us to move less and sit the majority of the day, which results in a huge tip of the seesaw towards a positive energy balance. However, what we often fail to realise is that the problem is not the problem itself; the problem is our *attitude* towards the problem. We must have a flexible mindset and learn to adjust to the modern environment so that we can make the most of everything on offer.

Life needs to be full of good habits day in, day out, and the only way to ensure you follow good habits is to create your own supportive environment. Whether it is for yourself, you and your family, or you and your partner, the same principles apply – you must eat healthy foods and you must move. That doesn't mean you can't enjoy the pleasures of life, you simply can't enjoy them all the time! For six out of seven days, you need to follow a structured plan that consists of home cooking and regular activity (see Part 2 of this book for suggestions). We are creatures of habit – we need some consistency and routine to ensure we succeed, but we also need some flexibility so that we don't get stuck in a rut, day in, day out.

'To do' lists

What is the best way to create a structured plan? You need to organise your day and use action plans. When we were children we were told what to do, which gave us discipline and routine, and kept us in line. As adults we need to do the same thing. The patients I've seen who lose weight most successfully are those who use 'to do' lists or 'structured day plans' every day. To put this into perspective, step into Stephanie's world.

When I first met Stephanie, she was a busy working mother of two, who struggled to stay on top of her work and look after her kids, and often found herself grabbing food on the run. To help Stephanie, I suggested she keep an ongoing list of things she needed to do each day. She preferred to do this electronically on her phone, but it really doesn't matter if you choose to do it on paper. I got her to include anything that popped into her head, even when she was on the go – walking, on the bus, watching television – whenever she remembered that she needed to do something, I got her to make a note of it so she didn't forget. It was a simple, effective task that gave her a huge sense of achievement and created a positive attitude. Having a successful routine in place also helped her to stop buying takeaway food.

A sample 'to do' list by Stephanie consisted of the following:

1. Scan letter to solicitor ☑
2. Email Peter about postage ☑
3. Wash and change bed sheets ☐
4. Meet with Sophie about move to new building ☑
5. Develop standard operating procedure for new staff members ☑
6. Sweep out garage ☐
7. Hose down balcony ☐
8. Drop chairs off to William ☐
9. Return books to library ☑
10. Email certificate to human resources ☑
11. Meet Jeff for game of squash ☑
12. Take out rubbish bins ☑
13. Source paint for bathroom ☐
14. Prepare tax documents ☐
15. Research secondary schools for Alex ☐
16. Analyse survey results ☑

17. Write up report of survey results ☐

18. Buy card and present for Thomas's birthday ☐

19. Write presentation for new intake of students ☐

At times your 'to do' list may seem quite overwhelming and you may find yourself adding more things to the list throughout a given day than you manage to complete, but that is okay. On other days you may well complete more things than you have added and feel a huge sense of achievement. Either way, you are succeeding if you update your 'to do' list every day and complete a structured daily plan first thing in the morning (see below). You must not let yourself feel down if the list never seems to be decreasing. That is not the point of the exercise – the point is for you to reflect on what you *have* achieved, so that you can give yourself a pat on the back, and to help you focus on what's important.

It doesn't matter what's on the list, it just matters that there is a list. Write this 'to do' list at the start of every day and tick off things or cross them out as you complete them.

Smartphone applications, such as Todoist, are fantastic for this sort of thing, and so are traditional notepads.

Ticking or crossing off tasks throughout the day gives you a sense of being rewarded and of satisfaction. It helps you develop confidence in yourself, and brings structure and routine into your life. You have to learn to praise yourself for doing the simple things in life. Once you have written down what needs to be done for the day, you can then write a plan for what you will do throughout the day (breaking it up into 15-minute, half-hour, or hour blocks). Again, this can be done electronically (perhaps in your work calendar, so that you can factor in any meetings you may have) or on a paper pad. A sample of one of Stephanie's structured day plans consisted of the following, which she would have put together the night before or first thing in the morning:

> 6–7 am: Wake up, shower, weigh myself, have breakfast, prepare lunch, hang out washing, leave for work.
>
> 7–8 am: Get bus to work. Write up 'to do' list for the day on the bus.
>
> 8–9 am: Send emails, do administration/paperwork.
>
> 9–9.30 am: Meet with Sophie regarding move to new building.
>
> 9.30–10 am: Team meeting.
>
> 10–12: Work on standard operating procedures for new staff members.
>
> 12–12.30 pm: Go outside and walk for 30 minutes (return books to library).
>
> 12.30–2 pm: Continue working on standard operating procedures for new staff members.
>
> 2–3 pm: Catch up on emails.

3–5.15 pm: Analyse results from survey.

5.15–5.30 pm: Travel to squash court.

5.30–6.30 pm: Play squash with Jeff.

6.30–7 pm: Pick up kids from Mum's.

7–7.15 pm: Drive home.

7.15–7.30 pm: With help from kids, take out rubbish bins, bring in washing and prepare dinner.

7.30–8 pm: Family dinner.

8–8.30 pm: Clean up kitchen with kids and make lunch for next day.

8.30–9.30 pm: Write in journal and relax.

9.30–10 pm: Prepare for bed.

10 pm: In bed.

You may notice that on this given day Stephanie didn't accomplish everything on her 'to do' list. It is rare that someone would, and some things may get out of sync on your structured day plan, and you run out of time or complete a task faster than you expected. In the case of the former, just carry the tasks across to the next day and complete them as you can. This breakdown of your day and type of plan gives you structure, a sense of achievement, and the positive attitude needed to achieve a healthy lifestyle.

De-cluttering

Often de-cluttering or parting with things that we don't need helps us to move on to the next chapter in our lives. If we continue to hold on to everything from our past, we don't allow ourselves to move on and break through to our new self. This can be an exceptionally hard thing for those who hoard. Remember, if you don't use it, it is better off going to someone who can make use of it. How do you make that distinction? Easy – if you haven't used it in six months or it has been through a season unused, then remove it. Don't think that just having some clothes in your wardrobe that are two sizes smaller will motivate you to get back to your former weight. That simply doesn't work and you are in the wrong frame of mind if you are thinking like that. The focus needs to be taken off body weight altogether and one way to do that is to remove old clothes. If you do get back to that weight and it is realistic to do so, you can then reward yourself by buying some new clothes to mark your accomplishments. De-cluttering your life goes a long way towards success on this journey.

An organised life

It doesn't matter how simple or extensive your 'to do' lists and structured day plans are, as long as they are effective and help keep your life organised. I have, though, had clients tell me that they think it's silly and they don't need to write things down.

One very stubborn client, Geoff, refused for months! But I persisted with him and I can honestly say that once he started to do this simple task, he started to get his life in order and to lose weight. Geoff became so fond of the organisational task that he began to colour-code everything into categories and suggest different templates that I could use with other clients!

Just as it worked for Geoff, it has worked for hundreds of other people I have helped. This is a task that you must persevere with until it becomes daily habit, and this applies to everyone (including those in senior management at large multinational companies). An organised life results in a healthy lifestyle, which results in a healthy body weight. And this is why you are here, right?

CHAPTER 6

EXERCISE AND REST

*'You only ever grow as a human being if
you're outside your comfort zone.'*
— Percy Cerutty

Movement, whether it is in the form of structured physical activity or incidental exercise, is an essential part of the recipe for a healthy lifestyle. Before the 1980s and all of the technological developments that started to take place, we didn't need gyms, as we got our exercise from walking to and from work and the shops, or playing outside. As I've said repeatedly — and I make no apology for it, as it's so important — the people who have successfully lost weight and kept it off long-term (more than five years), are those who eat a large volume of wholesome food and perform a lot of daily activity. And this doesn't mean you need to go to a gym every day. It just means you need to move – and move a lot.

Steps

The first thing to do is to actually see how much activity you are doing, which means going to a sports store or pharmacy, or jumping online, and buying a pedometer. It doesn't matter what kind. Pedometers start from as little as $5. These will more than likely register steps while you are sitting or swivelling on your office chair, but it doesn't matter, as this over-reporting of your activity level will be consistent every day. There can be as much as a 20 per cent error. So, if it says you are doing 10,000 steps per day, you may actually be only doing 8000 steps. The next step up in the range is a 'pedometer accelerometer' (starting from about $20), which uses slightly better technology and only measures real movement. For instance, you need to be moving for more than 8 steps or 3 seconds continuously for it to start recording. And then you have the 'accelerometer', which works on a tri-axial method of measurement, recording all types and forms of movement, including sitting time. These are expensive, and not necessary for general day-to-day use unless you can afford one and enjoy tracking everything in detail.

There is also an abundance of wearable technologies, apps, and specific health applications on smartphones that allow you to track everything you do, including movement (steps) and sitting time (such examples include Charity Miles and Strava). If you decide to get an external monitoring device separate from your phone, such as a 'pedometer' or 'pedometer accelerometer', you'll need to wear it for a week to work out your baseline activity level, and from there start increasing it.

Incidental activity

Experts say that 10,000 steps is a good goal for general heart health, so measure your daily steps with a pedometer and track your steps either electronically or on paper. Measuring steps, however, is not the be-all and end-all, as it doesn't take into consideration intensity of the exercise, and there are activities such as riding, swimming or resistance training where a pedometer just will not function. In my eyes this is not the point of a pedometer. You need to use a pedometer to measure your incidental activity only. For example, the time spent walking to and from the bus stop, walking up stairs, walking to the printer, or any other activity that is part of your general day.

Your incidental goal must be 10,000 steps per day, so if you are nowhere near this, work towards it gradually. Think about realistic long-term ways in which you can achieve this goal, as there is no point in adding routines that are not going to stick. Public transport usually adds a lot of steps to a person's day, as does parking further away from the workplace, so that you are forced to get steps in before and after leaving work. If you drive to your workplace, you must start getting there earlier, so that you can go for a much-needed walk before starting your day. A 20-minute walk equals approximately 2500 steps, so if you can incorporate that into your commute to and from the office, you've already done 5000 steps without even thinking about it.

Take a break

A break during your day has the benefit of improved productivity, as you can clear your head for a few minutes of the tasks you were doing, while going for a walk. Getting outdoors for a break during lunch, for example, means you will get the vitamin D that you need for not only healthy bones and the prevention of osteoporosis but also for a healthy weight and blood pressure. Yes, that's right, vitamin D is essential for a healthy lifestyle, as it helps promote weight loss and improve blood pressure in those with low vitamin D levels. And if you are not sure whether you have healthy vitamin D levels, have this tested by your doctor during winter, which is when you are more at risk. Again, the winter months are especially important to be wary of not getting enough Vitamin D.

The weight-loss plateau

Many people become incredibly frustrated when they reach a weight-loss plateau. Are you one of those people who has been going to the gym for months with no results? Or, perhaps, been eating healthier but still the weight won't shift? Are you one of those people who has reached a weight-loss plateau?

> Paul, a client of mine who had been progressing well with the Interval Weight Loss approach, suddenly stopped losing weight. He hit a standstill and couldn't understand why. But there was a reason for it. He hadn't changed his exercise routine since the start of his new lifestyle plan and his body had acclimatised to what he had been doing. It no longer saw it as a 'stress', by which I mean a challenge. He needed, therefore, to get out of his comfort zone and stop doing the same thing day in, day out. His body needed to be challenged for him to continue to see success.

This applies to everyone, not just Paul. Do you think an athlete would keep improving if they followed the same program all the time? Of course not! Do you think you are going to lose weight if you keep doing the same thing all the time? Absolutely not! Variety is the key – if you keep doing what you have always done, you will keep getting what you have always got.

Structured activity

So, what should you be doing? On top of your 10,000 incidental steps per day, there must be room for structured activity. If there's one thing in particular that you really like to do (for example, running or swimming), you must not do the same session every time. Even if it's a mixture of different sports and physical activity you are doing throughout the week, it must not be the same routines. It must vary all the time. You must keep your body guessing and stress it beyond its comfort zone. For example, if you're really diligent, you might go to yoga on Monday, the gym on Tuesday, have a run on Wednesday, go back to the gym on Thursday, to Pilates on Friday and to the pool on Saturday. Yes, you have variety in your routine, but if each of those sessions is the same routine each time, you are not going to reap the weight loss rewards. Sure, you will still get the heart health and other benefits associated with exercise, but you won't lose the weight you are trying to shift.

Next time you go to the gym, do a different routine. Next time you go for a run, go on a different route. Next time you go to yoga, go on a different day to trial a different class intensity. Ideally, you should roll the dice every morning when you wake up, and each number from 1–6 (allowing for your day off) should represent a different activity that is part of your weekly routine. This will add an extra benefit, of mixing up the days that you do each type of exercise.

For instance, it will mean that you won't go for your run or to yoga on the same day each week. This extra element of variety can often also be enough to jolt you out of your comfort zone so that your body doesn't know what activity to prepare itself for. And trust me, it usually does know.

So, from this day forward you must stop doing what you have always done. Go to the park, walk or run up some hills, go to the gym, play tennis, go hiking – it doesn't matter what it is, as long as it's not the same. Let the dice determine what you are going to do, so that you don't stick to the same daily routine. Every day should be different, and every week should be different.

Time-poor days

There are weeks when you are so strapped for time that you can't even think about, let alone fit in, some form of structured activity. In these situations, you must still devote time to exercise but you must adopt a different approach. Time-poor days are ideal for utilising high-intensity exercise where you work at high heart rates with reduced recovery for shorter periods of time. You might incorporate sprints or hills if you are running, and if you are swimming, you might incorporate sprint laps, different strokes, or even pool running. For example, you might complete a bout of exercise such as a sprint for 30 seconds at maximum intensity, have one minute rest, and then repeat. Twenty minutes is fine, and if you are working hard enough you won't be able to exercise for any longer. This will make all the difference in keeping a positive outlook. Remember, all sports are great – the key is to enjoy them so that you stick to them long-term.

The gym

I mentioned before that you don't need to go to a gym every day to achieve success. In saying this, the gym does provide a great platform for variety and can be mixed into your routine a few days a week. Resistance or weight training provides great benefits from a body composition point of view.

If you are female and don't like to go to a gym because you think it will bulk you up, rest assured this is not true. As females have very low testosterone counts, muscle gain is extremely difficult, but muscle toning (due to reduction in fat tissue) is likely. The gym offers a platform to stress and challenge your body in different ways. You can target your whole body and, most importantly, minimise any associated decrease in lean muscle mass associated with weight loss.

If you are interested in trying a gym, make sure to check out several in your area to ensure you find the one that best suits all of your needs. After all, you must feel comfortable in the environment you are exercising in. Nowadays, memberships also include free gym programs, so you know what exercise and weights you should be lifting. All you need to remember is not to do the same program for more than 2–4 weeks. If you are thinking about signing up with a gym, make sure it includes a free instructional written program, and that it changes at a minimum of every 2–4 weeks. Despite what they might try to tell you, you must listen to my advice and modify your program every 2–4 weeks. They may try to sign you up with a program that lasts 6–8 weeks and if this is the case, that gym is not for you!

Children

Time is a rare commodity when you are raising children. It can feel as if there is barely time for sleep, let alone time for you. However, this doesn't mean exercise should be neglected. Often it means you might just need to push the pram around the streets, or run around the oval while your kids train for their sport. You can still exercise with your children in sight. I've had lots of cases of people reporting success stories during the time they are raising their children as they are forced to change their way of life. For example, they can no longer sit on the couch in the afternoon or evening, as they either need to do something for their child or to take them some-where. And if it's sport you are taking them to, this often provides a great opportunity to do something yourself. This can range from taking your kids to the playground to taking them to sports training. There are also plenty of exercise classes for parents and kids to join together. This is what you should consider a 'created opportunity'. If it wasn't for having to take your kid outdoors or to sport, you might be sitting at home or still be in front of the computer at work. Think of every stage of your life as an opportunity for success.

Post-pregnancy

Your weight and body shape *can* return to how they were pre-pregnancy. Trust me! Try to get back into low-intensity activity as soon as you are able to (for example, pushing the pram around your local neighbourhood) and gradually progress back into high-intensity activity. It will take time, so be patient and don't forget that you're doing the most important job in the world – raising a child! Remember that fact every time you see an unrealistic photograph of a celebrity model who has bounced back into shape seemingly overnight.

Exercise myths

Just as there are common misconceptions surrounding different foods, there are also misconceptions surrounding exercise. And some of them seem to keep rebounding despite research proving them untrue.

Should I fast and exercise in the morning?

Some people think that fasting in the morning and exercising first thing increase how much fat they will burn, but you are not going to burn more fat because you are fasting. You will burn exactly the same amount of calories – and the number of calories will depend on the type of exercise, not the food, or lack of food, you may have had beforehand. So this means that you are no better off exercising in the morning, compared with in the evening. Exercise when it suits you!

Is low-intensity exercise better than high-intensity exercise for fat loss?

No! Your respiratory quotient (ratio of carbon dioxide expired to oxygen consumed) will determine the predominant energy source you will burn. If it is low-intensity exercise, you will be burning a higher percentage of fat and if you are doing high-intensity exercise you will be burning a higher percentage of carbohydrate, but with high-intensity exercise you are working at higher heart rates, which equates to a continuation of energy and fat stores being burned after exercise. Include a mixture of low- and high-intensity exercise, as this is important for heart health, variety and enjoyment.

Will a lot of crunches or sit-ups help me lose my tummy?

There is no such thing as spot-target fat reduction. You will only lose weight off your stomach if you are burning more energy than you are putting into it, and hence you will lose weight from your entire body. Unfortunately for males, the stomach can be the most stubborn area in which to see a difference; often it is the hips for females, as this is where they store the most fat. Sure, crunches or sit-ups (as with any core stomach exercise) will help develop muscle tone but only if you are doing enough exercise and burning sufficient calories to burn the fat off.

Will doing weights make me put on muscle or make me bigger?

No, as I've said, weights or resistance training will offer a variety of training for your exercise and physical activity routine, and help minimise any loss of lean muscle mass associated with weight loss. Females will not put on muscle with weights training but will instead tone muscle if they are burning adequate energy stores (as their muscle to fat ratio will increase, giving a leaner and more defined appearance). This will be the same for males if they are burning adequate energy stores (i.e. burning more energy than they are putting into their body). Muscle weighs more than fat, so you may find your weight plateauing after incorporating a weights program into your routine (this is especially relevant for males, who have higher testosterone levels than females and therefore are more likely to build muscle). An increase in your muscle to fat ratio is a good result and will help with long-term weight maintenance.

The importance of sleep

After all that exercise, sleep is one of the most important aspects of completing your journey to a healthy lifestyle. An improvement in your nutrition intake, and increase in your exercise output, should go a long way towards improving your sleep quality. You must aim to get 7–8 hours of sleep per night. Sleep quality is especially important, so it is best to do all you can to prevent insomnia. This means no caffeine (e.g. chocolate, cocoa, coffee or tea) within 4–6 hours of bed. I recommend 6 hours, to be certain. For example, if you go to bed at 10pm, you should have no further caffeine after 4pm. And despite what many people think, green tea is not caffeine-free. The only tea that is caffeine-free is herbal tea, which is based on herbal infusion from the leaves of the particular tree.

Alcohol will also disrupt your sleep quality, so if you choose to drink, as mentioned earlier keep it to 1 average-sized drink per day because we tend to fill our glasses quite high (which equates closely enough to 2 standard drinks), with a minimum of 2 alcohol-free days per week. Lastly, avoid eating 2 hours before bed. This allows adequate time for digestion before attempting to fall asleep.

Screen time

Dissociate television from the bedroom by ensuring you don't have one in there. This also applies to other screens, such as computers and phones. Don't use them before going to sleep and keep them well away from you while you sleep. They emit a blue wavelength of light, which disrupts circadian rhythms (the body clock) making it difficult to get to sleep. This blue light emission is detrimental in suppressing our melatonin levels, which have a role in signalling us to go to sleep. These devices are in essence telling our brain that it is daytime and not time to sleep.

Your bedroom is not a place for screens and work, so, again, it must be completely dissociated from those sorts of activities.

The next thing to consider is your bed quality. Do you have a good-quality bed? If so, you can ignore what I am about to say. You spend approximately one third of your day in bed – this is much more than we would spend commuting in our car. So, invest in a good-quality bed and pillow. Sleep is one of the most important aspects of your health, so don't be scared to spend a few dollars on it. It is much more important to buy a decent bed than to buy some commodity you barely use and often have paid more for.

When we discussed the art of mindful eating before, we focused on supper time and ensuring you partake in activities that are constructive. Another one of those constructive activities, believe it or not, is sleep! The earlier you go to bed, the better. Especially if you have forgotten what it feels like to wake up without an alarm clock each day. It is much better to go to bed early and wake up naturally than it is to go to bed late and wake up to an alarm clock. You will feel fresher all day, as you are not waking up during one of your sleep cycles.

If you are one of those people who struggles to get to sleep at night, this should improve with an increase and/or change in your exercise or physical activity program. Practising relaxation techniques such as yoga and meditation before bed can also help. If you are unsure of what to do, watch a video, listen to a recording online or use a smartphone application such as Silva Method. These types of activity teach you to take control over your body, which you can then apply to all facets of your life.

So now you're rested and re-energised, you're losing weight and keeping it off, when will you know if you've been successful long-term?

Long-term success

It is one thing to lose the weight but it's another to keep it off long-term. You should consider yourself successful when you have lost weight and kept it off for 5 years (give or take a couple of kilograms). Unfortunately, the majority of weight-loss research is not conducted for this long, as interventions and follow-up (especially prospective, randomised, controlled trials that are considered the gold standard of clinical research) are usually only over 2–3 years at the most. However, since I have been fortunate enough to be at my current workplace for nearly a decade, I have witnessed a lot of people succeed well past this 5-year time period. Some of the people we recruit for our research come from the institution where I work (which has approximately 60,000 staff and students) or our neighbouring institution at Royal Prince Alfred Hospital. This has meant that I often bump into people I have helped many years down the track, and they proudly show and tell me that they have nearly hit, or already hit, the 5-year mark of successfully keeping the weight off.

Many of the people I have met on this journey have asked whether I have any meal suggestions that I could share with them. So, read Part 2 of this book for some delicious recipes and meal plans to inspire you!

PART 2

CREATIVE COOKING

This section is not intended to be a traditional cookbook. In modern times, technology places food ideas at your fingertips; social media platforms ensure there is no shortage of recipes and, in fact, in many instances there are too many versions of recipes (and I will get to why, later). I am not a chef and do not claim to be one, but cooking is a wonderful and fulfilling aspect of a healthy lifestyle, as it encourages us to appreciate and enjoy the food we eat. Importantly, it can be basic enough so that anyone can cook, whatever your level of experience.

I was lucky enough to complete certificates in commercial cookery as part of my tertiary education studies, which allowed me to practise the art of inventive cooking in substituting healthier alternatives for ingredients. The great thing is, creativity can be applied to cooking in many different ways, and the recipes that follow are intended to demonstrate just that. They support the basic concept that I have promoted throughout this book – that is, wherever possible, you should eat food based on raw ingredients rather than relying on pre-packaged or pre-made food. There are times when convenience foods can play a role, but cooking can just as easily be executed using raw ingredients as pre-made ingredients. For example, making a pasta sauce from scratch is simple and it will be more nutritious and delicious than pre-made sauce from a jar.

To return to my earlier point about the many instances where traditional recipes have been altered with endless substitute ingredients, I am specifically referring to 'treat' foods. A treat food should be a treat (no more than once per week!). If you are worried about the ingredients in a particular food, this means you are having it far too often. If you follow this essential lifestyle principle, you can enjoy the food (whether it is at home or when eating out) without having a guilty conscience, or worrying about what other people think. This means that when you are baking a cake, a chocolate brownie, a caramel slice, or whatever your favourite treat food may be, you can cook it in its traditional form without having to feel guilty because you're only having it once a week. If you prefer to substitute ingredients in a home-cooked recipe, this is, of course, also fine, but only if your palate enjoys the revised version. For example, you might reduce the quantity of oil used in a recipe, or substitute butter for oil, as in the carrot cake slice recipe later in the book.

Once you have all the staples in your kitchen cupboard, cooking should be easy and enjoyable and, as a bonus, will save you money. It can be even easier if you have children, as they can be part of the cooking experience, which will teach them important life skills and ensure they are domesticated when they're older. The great thing is, even if you make a mistake and your meal is a disaster, this is something you can learn from and the dish is bound to taste better next time around. I am also a big believer in not over-complicating things in the kitchen, given the time-poor schedule many of us have. This means choosing recipes that can be followed easily and have a lot of flexibility to ensure your meal is appetising every time.

STORE CUPBOARD ESSENTIALS

Keep a good supply of these foods in your kitchen, and when they start to run low, make sure you add them to your shopping list before they run out completely. Don't be overwhelmed by the following list as these are staples that will last for a long time. And if you're a beginner or have few cooking skills, they can be accumulated over time, as your confidence with cooking develops.

Oils: olive or canola oil (all of the recipes reference olive oil but canola oil can also be used)

Dried goods: unsalted dry-roasted or raw nuts (almonds, walnuts, cashews), a variety of seeds (sunflower, flaxseed, pumpkin, sesame), wholemeal flour (plain and self-raising), dried breadcrumbs, pasta (including wholemeal), rice (basmati, brown rice), rolled oats, couscous, dried pulses (lentils, chickpeas, split peas), sugar

Tinned food: tomatoes, chickpeas, lentils, a variety of beans, corn, beetroot, pineapple, tuna and salmon, tomato paste (always opt for low or no added salt)

Condiments: soy sauce, vegetable stock, honey, lemon and lime juice (as a back-up to fresh lemon or limes), maple syrup, tahini paste, nut butter, jarred garlic, ginger and chilli (jarred with vinegar only, and as a back-up to fresh garlic, ginger or chilli)

Dried herbs and spices: black pepper, chilli flakes, oregano, coriander, basil, thyme, turmeric, cumin, mixed herbs, mustard seeds

Long-lasting vegetables: brown onions, sweet potato, ginger, garlic

Perishables: no-fat or low-fat milk, yoghurt, eggs and wholegrain bread

Frozen food: berries, edamame, frozen vegetables

Beverages: green tea, herbal teas

Fresh herbs and spices

I believe everyone should grow the bare essentials when it comes to herbs and spices, even if you live in an apartment. It doesn't take much work, and just a little maintenance will go a long way to ensuring you have fresh produce at your fingertips. In addition, it will save you money, as one of the biggest wastes of produce is when we buy fresh herbs from the supermarket and only use a small quantity. Growing herbs is also a great project for children, as it gives them responsibility, and a sense of achievement and of contribution when they see the great results.

The staples include basil, parsley, oregano, thyme, rosemary, chives, spring onions, chilli and coriander. Coriander and some varieties of chilli can be challenging to grow but the others will usually thrive with some sunlight, water and good nutrient soil (don't buy cheap potting mix, as it will ensure failure!).

Talk to the people at your local nursery – they'll be happy to help you with your selections. Start small and expand your collection of herbs as you begin to understand what works best in your home environment. For those who develop a green thumb, the opportunities are endless. Tomatoes are wonderful to grow at home and you will notice a much sweeter flavour in your home-grown produce than in anything you can buy from the supermarket. Rainbow spinach is also a very easily grown leafy vegetable that is great to have on hand.

SUGGESTED MEAL PLAN

The purpose of these weekly meal plans is to give you examples of how to plan your day. Again, your main focus should be on eating a larger quantity of food in the earlier part of the day and tapering off during the afternoon, so that dinner is your smallest meal. If you are cooking for the family, serve yourself a smaller meal at dinner time and aim to have leftovers that you can use for lunch the next day. As I've said, the evening meal should be served on a bread and butter plate or in a rice bowl.

The key thing to remember is that all food should be eaten away from technological distraction. This will ensure you focus on chewing properly and, more importantly, allow you to enjoy the food itself. And remember to eat before hunger pangs set in. Have a water bottle with you at work or home, and remember to sip on it continuously throughout the day.

All of the recipes in this book can be utilised in any of your weekly plans.

DAY 1: MONDAY

Breakfast
2 poached, soft-boiled or fried eggs on 2 slices of wholegrain
    toast, with avocado
Milk-based coffee
1 cup (250 ml) water

Morning tea
No-fat or low-fat yoghurt (natural or flavoured)
1 cup (250 ml) water

Lunch
Pumpkin couscous (see page 142)
1 cup (250 ml) water

Afternoon tea
Celery or carrot sticks with beetroot dip or beetroot hummus
    (see pages 167 and 168)
1 cup (250 ml) water

Dinner
Spicy meatball and broccoli pasta (see page 138)

DAY 2: TUESDAY

Breakfast

Oats with cinnamon, yoghurt and berries on top

Milk-based coffee

1 cup (250 ml) water

Morning tea

1 slice of wholegrain toast with peanut butter or jam

1 cup (250 ml) water

Lunch

Salad made from rocket, avocado, cherry or grape tomatoes,
    tinned tuna or salmon, and a drizzle of olive oil

Wholegrain crackers

1 cup (250 ml) water

Afternoon tea

Handful of unsalted dry-roasted or raw nuts

Piece of fruit

1 cup (250 ml) water

Dinner

Greek-style lamb sliders (see page 175)

DAY 3: WEDNESDAY

Breakfast
2 slices of wholegrain toast with avocado
No-fat or low-fat yoghurt (natural or flavoured)
1 cup (250 ml) water

Morning tea
Milk-based coffee
Piece of fruit
1 cup (250 ml) water

Lunch
Chicken and salad wholegrain sandwich (this can be bought
    from a sandwich shop if it is made on the spot so that you
    can control what goes in it)
1 cup (250 ml) water

Afternoon tea
Boiled egg with a slice of wholegrain toast
1 cup (250 ml) water

Dinner
Japanese-inspired salmon (see page 157)

DAY 4: THURSDAY

Breakfast

Breakfast smoothie (see page 113)

Slice of wholegrain toast with honey or jam

1 cup (250 ml) water

Morning tea

Milk-based coffee

1 cup (250 ml) water

Lunch

Tinned tuna on 2 slices of wholegrain bread or toast

1 cup (250 ml) water

Afternoon tea

Handful of mixed nuts and seeds

1 cup (250 ml) water

Dinner

Roast lamb with roast sweet potato, pumpkin and zucchini
(personal preference will determine how long you cook your
leg of lamb, but remember that lamb is already tender so try
not to overcook it)

DAY 5: FRIDAY

Breakfast

No-fat or low-fat yoghurt (natural or flavoured)

Piece of fruit

1 cup (250 ml) water

Morning tea

Milk-based coffee

Handful of nuts and seeds

1 cup (250 ml) water

Lunch

Tuna, or salmon, and salad wholegrain sandwich (this can be
bought from a sandwich shop if it is made on the spot so
that you can control what goes in it)

1 cup (250 ml) water

Afternoon tea

Chopped carrot and celery sticks with peanut butter

1 cup (250 ml) water

Dinner

Barbecued or grilled steak with green salad

DAY 6: SATURDAY

Breakfast

2 eggs with avocado on 2 slices of wholegrain toast

Tea or milk-based coffee

1 cup (250 ml) water

Morning tea

Breakfast smoothie (see page 113)

1 cup (250 ml) water

Lunch

Grilled beef, eggplant and pomegranate salad (see page 129)

1 cup (250 ml) water

Afternoon tea

Natural yoghurt with a sprinkle of ground cinnamon

1 cup (250 ml) water

Dinner

Takeaway or dining out – this can be classified as your 'treat'
meal and therefore no restrictions apply

DAY 7: SUNDAY

Breakfast

2-egg omelette (including diced capsicum, spring onions, parsley, rainbow spinach and mushrooms) with 2 slices of wholegrain toast

Tea or milk-based coffee

1 cup (250 ml) water

Morning tea

Fruit bowl with berries, chopped seasonal fruit, no-fat or low-fat yoghurt, and ground cinnamon sprinkled on top

Milk-based coffee

1 cup (250 ml) water

Lunch

Roast chicken and salad from takeaway shop (remove skin from chicken)

1 cup (250 ml) water

Afternoon tea

1 slice of wholegrain toast with your spread of choice

1 cup (250 ml) water

Dinner

Pumpkin, tomato and ginger soup (see page 125)

1 row of dark chocolate

BREAKFAST

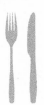

BREAKFAST SMOOTHIE

This smoothie, with no-fat or low-fat milk, gives you a serve of dairy and a highly absorbed source of calcium. You can add all sorts of ingredients to a smoothie – for example, try including 30 grams (a small handful) of nuts in place of the rolled oats. Fluids are not as filling as whole foods; smoothies mustn't be an addition to a meal but, rather, a meal option when you're time-poor or a snack between meals.

Serves 1

½ cup (75 g) blueberries (fresh or frozen)
2 heaped tablespoons low-fat frozen yoghurt
2 tablespoons rolled oats
½ banana
1 cup (250 ml) 100% fruit juice or no-fat or low-fat milk
ice cubes
½ teaspoon ground cinnamon (optional)

1. Mix the ingredients in a blender and enjoy!

BANANA AND BLUEBERRY PANCAKES

This is an exceptionally easy and nutritious breakfast – it's great for weekends, when you can really take the time to enjoy it. It is also gluten free, making it a delicious option for those who are coeliac and on a gluten-free diet.

Serves 4

1 cup (90 g) rolled oats
2 bananas, mashed
2 eggs
1 cup (150 g) blueberries
olive oil spray
sliced mango (optional)

1. Place the oats in a food processor or blender, and mix until they are the consistency of flour. Add the mashed banana, eggs and ¾ of the blueberries, and mix (in the food processor or blender) to form a batter.
2. Heat a large frying pan over medium heat and spray with olive oil.
3. Pour small quantities of the mixture into the frying pan (working in batches of roughly 4 pancakes in the pan at a time) and cook for a couple of minutes or until bubbles begin to form on the surface of each pancake. Flip each pancake when light bubbling is evident, and cook for a further couple of minutes or until golden and cooked through. Put them

on a plate and cover to keep warm while you cook the remaining pancakes (the amount of pancakes this mixture makes will depend on their size).

4. Serve the pancakes with the remaining blueberries, and mango, if desired.

EGGS WITH CRUMBLED FETA AND SMOKED SALMON

It is a misconception that eggs increase your blood cholesterol level. They can be enjoyed every day of the week, in combination with a healthy food intake that is low in 'bad' fats and high in 'good' fats. This simple recipe is a good example of how to use them.

Serves 1

2 eggs
¼ avocado
juice of ¼ lemon
2 slices wholegrain bread, toasted
2 slices smoked salmon
1 tablespoon crumbled feta cheese

1. Place the eggs in a saucepan of cold water and bring to the boil. Once the water is boiling, remove the pan from the heat and leave the eggs in the hot water for 4–5 minutes, depending on how you like them (4 minutes will give you a softer yolk). Drain, then submerge the eggs in cold water to stop the cooking process. When they're cool enough to handle, peel the eggs and slice thickly.
2. Scoop the avocado flesh into a bowl, add the lemon juice and mash with a fork. Spread over the toasted bread, then layer on the smoked salmon and egg.
3. Sprinkle the feta over the top and serve.

Tip: You can check whether eggs are fresh by placing them in a bowl of water. If they float, they are old; if they sink, they are fresh. Store them in the fridge.

SPICY MIDDLE EASTERN BREAKFAST EGGS

This is a wonderful, flavoursome dish that will add variety to your weekend breakfast.

Serves 4

1 tablespoon olive oil, for cooking

2 garlic cloves, crushed

½ red onion, thinly sliced, or 1 large handful of chopped spring onions

1 red chilli, finely chopped (seeds can be removed, or kept for extra heat)

2 teaspoons hot paprika

2 teaspoons ground cumin

½ teaspoon ground coriander

1 x 400 g tin tomatoes

½ red capsicum, seeds and membrane removed, sliced

4 eggs

sprinkle of fresh coriander, chopped finely, to garnish

1. Heat the olive oil in a large frying pan over medium heat. Add the garlic and onion or spring onions and cook for three minutes or until softened.
2. Add the chilli, paprika, cumin and ground coriander and stir until fragrant.
3. Add the tomatoes and capsicum and cook, stirring frequently, for 10 minutes.

4. Using a wooden spoon, create four large indents in the mixture. Crack an egg into each hole, and do not stir the mixture.

5. Reduce the heat to low, and cook for 8–10 minutes or until the eggs are to your liking. Sprinkle with fresh coriander and serve.

Tip: Some supermarkets stock jarred garlic, in its natural form – that is, it will only contain garlic (usually around 88%) and vinegar, and 1 teaspoon is equivalent to 1 clove of garlic. Steer clear of the jarred garlic that contains a mixture of other ingredients. Remember that the jarred garlic is only a back-up; if you can, keep a bulb of fresh garlic on hand – it will store well for a while. Use a garlic press to crush the cloves, to minimise the garlicky smell you get on your fingers if you chop it up by hand.

SOUPS AND SALADS

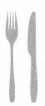

ROASTED SWEET POTATO SOUP

Sweet potato is lower in the glycemic index than potato and is therefore a suitable switch in many recipes. Being lower in glycemic index means the food is digested, absorbed and metabolised more slowly, which keeps you feeling full and satisfied for longer. As a variation on the recipe, try adding green peas to the soup. They will serve the dual purpose of bringing extra flavour and sweetness and lowering the glycemic index.

Serves 2

1 large brown onion, roughly chopped
2 large sweet potatoes (about 1 kg), diced
2 carrots, diced
2 garlic cloves, crushed
1 teaspoon coriander seeds
olive oil spray
1½ cups (375 ml) vegetable stock
chopped flat-leaf parsley or coriander, to garnish

1. Preheat the oven to 160°C.
2. Place the onion, sweet potato, carrot and garlic in a large baking dish. Sprinkle the coriander seeds over them and lightly spray with olive oil.
3. Bake for 40 minutes or until the vegetables are tender (check with a fork – it should go in easily).

4. Blend the vegetables and stock in a blender (or with a stick blender) until smooth and well mixed.

5. Pour the soup into a large saucepan and warm it through. Ladle into bowls and serve topped with parsley or coriander.

PUMPKIN, TOMATO AND GINGER SOUP

This simple soup is a great example of how homegrown tomatoes can make all the difference to the flavour of a dish. This is a meal you can make in large batches and then freeze in individual containers for use throughout the week.

Serves 6–8

700 g ripe tomatoes
1 kg pumpkin (any variety), peeled and cut into, approximately, 2 cm pieces
3 brown onions, chopped
2 teaspoons ground ginger
1 litre vegetable or chicken stock (see page 126)
freshly ground black pepper
chopped flat-leaf parsley or chives, to garnish

1. Cut a cross in the base of the tomatoes and place in a heatproof bowl. Cover with boiling water and leave for about a minute until the skins start to peel away. Remove from the water and, when cool enough to handle, slip off the skins.
2. Place the tomatoes, pumpkin, onion and ginger in a large saucepan, then pour in the stock and enough water to cover the vegetables. Bring to the boil, then reduce the heat and simmer for 15 minutes, or until the pumpkin is tender.
3. Puree in a blender (or with a stick blender) and season with pepper to taste.
4. Ladle into bowls and garnish with parsley or chives.

HOMEMADE CHICKEN STOCK

Homemade stock is always going to be best, and it's so easy to make. Place a chicken carcass (maybe the leftovers from a roast) in a large saucepan or stockpot and cover generously with water. Bring to the boil, then reduce the heat to low and simmer, covered, for 1 hour, skimming any froth from the top. Add a variety of vegetables, herbs and spices (such as carrots, celery, onion, ginger, garlic, parsley, thyme, dill and black pepper) and continue to simmer for 2–4 hours, stirring occasionally (the longer you leave it to simmer, the more intense the flavour will be). Strain the entire contents of the saucepan to remove the solids. Refrigerate the stock for 12–24 hours. During this time the fat will rise to the top and set, making it easy to remove and discard. The stock will keep in the fridge for up to 4 days or in the freezer for up to 3 months.

What is in pre-made liquid stock we buy off the shelves? Pre-made stocks are generally prepared in a similar way to the above, although they often include additional ingredients such as sugar, yeast extract or vegetable extract powders. Always opt for a low-sodium (salt) variety and check the ingredients list. Some suitable brands include Campbell's and Essential Cuisine.

SWEET POTATO AND LENTIL SOUP

This is great to make in large batches for meals throughout the week. It also freezes really well. I suggest using chicken stock, for a greater depth of flavour, if you don't need the soup to be vegetarian. Also, replace sweet potato with pumpkin if preferred.

Serves 4

1 cup (200 g) red lentils
1 litre vegetable stock
1 tablespoon olive oil
1 teaspoon ground turmeric
1 teaspoon ground coriander
1 teaspoon ground cumin
2 teaspoons yellow or brown mustard seeds
1 tablespoon grated ginger
1 large sweet potato, grated
1 spoonful of no-fat yoghurt, to serve
1 teaspoon flat-leaf parsley or coriander, chopped finely, to garnish

1. Combine the lentils, stock and olive oil in a large saucepan and bring to the boil. Reduce the heat and simmer for 12 minutes, stirring regularly.
2. Add the ground spices, mustard seeds and ginger and simmer for a further 10 minutes or until fragrant.

3. Add the sweet potato and simmer for 30 minutes or until the mixture has thickened. Serve with a dollop of yoghurt, and garnish with fresh herbs such as flat-leaf parsley or coriander.

GRILLED BEEF, EGGPLANT AND POMEGRANATE SALAD

The success of this salad largely depends on the quality of the beef. Start with an appropriate cut, such as rump or porterhouse, trim any visible fat and, most importantly, let it rest before you serve it. Resting allows the juices to be redistributed through the meat, making it more tender and juicy.

Serves 4

olive oil, for cooking
½ eggplant, thinly sliced, and sliced again so the pieces are
   bite-sized
4 spring onions (1/2 cup), chopped
½ red chilli, finely chopped
300 g beef steak, such as rump or porterhouse
75 g vermicelli noodles
large handful of bean sprouts
3 tablespoons lime juice mixed with 1 teaspoon sugar (any type)
125 g cherry or grape tomatoes, halved
seeds from 1/2 pomegranate
basil or flat-leaf parsley leaves, to garnish

1. Heat a heavy frying pan or cast-iron grill plate over medium heat and drizzle with olive oil. Add the eggplant and cook for a few minutes, then add the spring onions and chilli and continue to cook until the eggplant is lightly browned and

soft. Transfer the eggplant mixture to a bowl, and clean out the pan.

2. Add another drizzle of olive oil to the pan or grill plate, add the beef and cook over medium heat, turning once, for 3–5 minutes or until cooked to your taste. Place the steak on a plate, cover tightly with foil and leave for a few minutes.

3. Meanwhile, cover the noodles with boiling water and set aside for a few minutes to soften. Drain in a strainer and run cold water over them.

4. Cut the steak into small strips and add to the eggplant mixture, along with the noodles and bean sprouts. Add lime juice mixture, tomatoes and pomegranate seeds and gently toss. Garnish with basil or parsley leaves and serve.

GREEK SALAD

This salad is just made to be eaten outside in the sunshine, preferably with some lamb cutlets hot off the barbecue. Quick to assemble, with easy-to-find ingredients, it's the perfect meal to share with friends.

Serves 4–6

3 Lebanese cucumbers, skins removed and roughly chopped
1 small red onion, sliced
1 red capsicum, seeds and membrane removed, roughly chopped
1 green capsicum, seeds and membrane removed, roughly chopped
250 g ripe tomatoes, roughly chopped
handful of Kalamata olives (or any variety you like)
150 g Greek feta cheese, roughly chopped
2 teaspoons dried oregano
sprinkle of dried chilli flakes (optional)
1 tablespoon of olive oil

1. Combine the cucumber, onion, capsicum, tomato and olives in a large serving bowl.
2. Sprinkle the oregano and chilli flakes (if using) over the top.
3. Scatter the feta over the top, drizzle with a tablespoon of olive oil, and serve.

POACHED CHICKEN SALAD

Poaching chicken is a wonderful, healthy alternative to roasting chicken. Roasting chicken results in the fat and oils from the skin cooking through the chicken; poaching chicken, as in this recipe, results in the same tender, juicy meat by absorbing the flavours of the coriander and lime, without the added fat.

Serves 4

1 lime, halved
large handful of coriander leaves, chopped
4 chicken breast fillets, thickly sliced
2 large handfuls of baby spinach leaves
125 g cherry or grape tomatoes, halved
150 g vermicelli noodles
2 Lebanese cucumbers, shaved

1. Thinly slice one of the lime halves and place in a large deep frying pan with half the coriander and 1 cup (250 ml) water. Bring to the boil over high heat, then reduce the heat to low, add the chicken and poach for about 10 minutes or until cooked through.
2. Remove from the heat and strain. Set the chicken aside to cool.
3. Cover the noodles with boiling water and set aside for a few minutes to soften. Drain in a strainer and run cold water over them.

4. Place the noodles in a serving bowl, add the baby spinach, tomatoes, cucumber and the remaining coriander and gently toss. Add the chicken, then squeeze the remaining lime juice over the top and serve.

Tip: Chickens have bacteria present on their surface that can penetrate deep into the flesh, as they have a less dense surface than animals such as sheep or cows. Therefore, the inner meat of chicken needs to be cooked right through and no pink should be evident.

MAIN MEALS

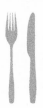

SPICY MEATBALLS

It's worth making a big batch of these meatballs to have on hand. Serve with a homemade tomato sauce, toss through a pasta dish (see spicy meatball and broccoli pasta recipe on page 138), or just enjoy them with a simple green salad. Leftovers are terrific for lunch the next day.

Makes 12–15 (4 servings)

1 egg
3 tablespoons grated cheddar
small handful of rocket, finely chopped
3 tablespoons almond meal
2 garlic cloves, crushed
1 teaspoon dried oregano
pinch of freshly ground black pepper
½ teaspoon chilli flakes, or to taste
450 g lean beef mince
1 tablespoon olive oil

1. Mix the egg, cheese, rocket, almond meal, garlic, oregano, pepper and chilli flakes in a bowl. Add the beef and mix with your hands until combined. Form into 12–15 meatballs.
2. Heat olive oil in a large frying pan over medium heat. Add the meatballs and cook for 8 minutes, or until browned all over and cooked through.

Tip: Veal can be used instead of beef.

SPICY MEATBALL AND BROCCOLI PASTA

Apart from tasting great, broccoli is packed full of antioxidants which remove 'free radicals' from the bloodstream, helping to protect the body from illnesses such as cancer. Paired with the meatballs, it makes a really satisfying pasta dish that you can have on the table in less than 20 minutes.

Serves 2

150 g pasta (any variety, preferably wholemeal)
2 tablespoons olive oil
150 g meatballs (see spicy meatballs recipe on page 137), cut
    into bite-sized pieces
½ garlic clove, finely chopped
¾ cup (60 g) broccoli florets
2 pinches of chilli flakes or finely chopped chilli, or to taste
small handful of flat-leaf parsley, chopped
freshly ground black pepper

1. Cook the pasta according to the packet instructions until al dente.
2. Meanwhile, heat 1 tablespoon olive oil in a frying pan over medium heat, add the garlic and broccoli florets, and cook for 5 minutes. Add the meatballs and warm them through with the garlic and broccoli florets for a couple of minutes.

3. Drain the pasta and add to the pan with the remaining olive oil. Sprinkle the chilli, parsley and pepper over the top and toss to mix. Serve with an extra grind of pepper, if desired.

ANGEL HAIR PASTA WITH SEAFOOD AND TOMATOES

Pasta is very low in fat and energy – it is the pasta sauce that can stack on the fat and calorie content of the meal, so it's always better to opt for a tomato-based sauce rather than high-fat creamy or cheesy sauces.

Serves 4

450 g assorted seafood (white fish fillets, mussels and raw
    prawns)
⅓ cup (80 ml) olive oil
2 garlic cloves, finely chopped
750 g ripe roma tomatoes or similar, roughly chopped
small handful of flat-leaf parsley, chopped, plus extra to garnish
freshly ground black pepper
300 g angel hair pasta, or spaghetti

1. Preheat the oven to 180°C.
2. Cut the fish into bite-sized pieces, clean and debeard the mussels, and peel and devein the prawns.
3. In a large casserole dish, combine the olive oil, garlic, tomatoes, parsley and a couple of pinches of pepper. Cover with a lid, then place in the oven and bake for 10 minutes.
4. Season the fish fillets with pepper, then add to the casserole dish and cook for another 10 minutes.
5. Add the mussels and prawns to the dish and bake for another 10 minutes. The mussels should open and the

prawns turn opaque. Discard any mussels that do
not open.

6. Meanwhile, cook the pasta according to the packet
   instructions until al dente.

7. Drain the pasta. Add it to the seafood mixture and gently
   toss to combine. Garnish with extra parsley and serve.

Tip: Wholemeal pasta has roughly twice the fibre content of
regular pasta. Why not give it a try? And always accompany
pasta-based meals with a side salad – the salad should fill half
of your plate or bowl.

PUMPKIN COUSCOUS

Couscous is a light, fluffy grain alternative to rice. It is usually steamed separately and served on the side, but this dish is another great way of having it. Try substituting other grains that are lower on the glycemic index, such as brown rice or pearl barley.

Serves 2

225 g pumpkin (any variety), peeled and cut into 2 cm cubes
½ beetroot, peeled and cut into 2 cm cubes
½ cup (125 ml) vegetable stock or water
½ cup (100 g) couscous
1 tablespoon olive oil
¼ red onion, finely chopped
2 tablespoons lemon juice
3 tablespoons finely chopped flat-leaf parsley, plus extra to
   serve

1. Place the pumpkin, beetroot and stock or water in a medium saucepan and bring to the boil. Cook for 5 minutes or until the vegetables are tender. Remove the pan from the heat and add the couscous. Cover and set aside for 3 minutes – the couscous will absorb the liquid. Fluff up the couscous with a fork.
2. Meanwhile, heat the olive oil in a small frying pan over

medium–low heat, add the onion and cook for 5–10 minutes or until softened and caramelised. Add the lemon juice and parsley during the last minute of cooking.

3. Gently toss the onion and couscous together, then sprinkle with extra parsley and serve.

Tip: This is a great meal to make in large batches and enjoy for lunch throughout the week.

MARINATED LAMB SKEWERS WITH GREEK YOGHURT

Lamb is extremely flavoursome and a good substitute for beef.
It works particularly well with Greek flavours, such as yoghurt,
oregano and lemon, making these skewers hard to resist.
Try them at your next barbecue.

Serves 2

100 g Greek yoghurt

½ garlic clove, crushed

1½ teaspoons dried oregano

½ teaspoon finely grated lemon zest

400 g boneless leg lamb, trimmed of fat and cut into
    4 cm cubes

½ green capsicum, seeds and membrane removed, cut into
    4 cm pieces

½ red capsicum, seeds and membrane removed, cut into
    4 cm pieces

½ red onion, cut into thin wedges

2 teaspoons olive oil

Greek salad (see page 131), to serve

1. In a glass bowl, mix the yoghurt, garlic, oregano and lemon
   zest. Transfer about ⅛ cup (2 tablespoons) to a separate
   bowl, add the lamb and coat it in the yoghurt mixture. Cover
   and chill in the fridge for a minimum of 30 minutes.

2. If you are using bamboo or wooden skewers, soak them in water for about 20 minutes before threading on the ingredients. This will stop the skewers burning during cooking.

3. Thread the lamb, capsicum and onion alternately onto the skewers.

4. Preheat a barbecue grill or cast-iron hot plate and drizzle with the olive oil. Place the skewers on it and cook, turning occasionally, for 5 minutes or until golden and cooked to your liking.

5. Serve the skewers with the remaining yoghurt mixture and Greek salad.

Tip: The surface of lamb and beef is often contaminated with pathogens; however, the meat is dense and the bacteria are unable to penetrate from the surface into the flesh. Therefore, these meats do not need to be cooked all the way through.

VEGETARIAN BURGERS

This is a good way to add variety to the weekly menu but still include a common family favourite – the hamburger! Beans offer wonderful flavour when accompanied by fresh herbs, and this recipe is a great alternative to the traditional beef burger. Adding more curry paste to the recipe gives a greater spice hit.

Makes 4

1 x 420 g tin five bean mix, drained and rinsed
1 x 300 g tin butter beans, drained and rinsed
1 cup (70 g) fresh breadcrumbs
1 tablespoon Thai curry paste
1 egg, lightly beaten
3 tablespoons chopped coriander
2 tablespoons lemon juice
freshly ground black pepper
2 tablespoons olive oil
4 pumpkin or grain-seed rolls, lightly toasted
large handful of rocket and baby spinach leaves
125 g cherry or grape tomatoes, chopped

1. Place all the beans in a food processor or blender, and pulse until the beans are roughly chopped.
2. Combine ½ cup (35 g) breadcrumbs, the curry paste, egg, coriander, lemon juice and a pinch of pepper in a bowl. Add the beans and mix well with your hands.

3. Form the mixture into four large patties and lightly coat in the remaining breadcrumbs, shaking off the excess.
4. Heat the olive oil in a large frying pan over medium heat. Add the patties and cook for 3–4 minutes each side or until golden brown and cooked through.
5. Fill the rolls with the patties, rocket and spinach, and chopped tomatoes.

Tip: If you like, double the recipe and make extra patties to freeze for eating another time. Separate them with plastic wrap, so you can easily remove them individually, then store in an airtight container in the freezer.

CHICKPEA AND ALMOND PANCAKES WITH SPICED SWEET POTATO

You can adapt the ingredients below to suit your palate. For instance, almonds have quite a distinct flavour and you may prefer to leave them out and increase the quantity of chickpeas, or replace the almonds with brown rice flour. You could also try adding some chia seeds. The difference between yellow and brown mustard seeds is the heat. Yellow (or white) mustard seeds are the mildest, while brown seeds are much spicier. Just use what works for you.

Serves 4

Greek yoghurt, to serve

Chickpea and almond pancakes
1 cup (200 g) tinned chickpeas
¾ cup (120 g) almonds
½ teaspoon bicarbonate of soda
1 teaspoon yellow or brown mustard seeds
½ teaspoon ground turmeric
olive oil spray

Spiced sweet potato
1 medium sweet potato, cut into small cubes
2 teaspoons olive oil
1 small brown onion, sliced

1 teaspoon yellow or brown mustard seeds

1 green or red chilli, seeded and finely chopped

2 garlic cloves, finely chopped

2 teaspoons grated ginger

½ teaspoon ground turmeric

1. To make the pancake batter, blend the chickpeas, almonds and 100 ml water in a high-powered blender, until smooth. Add the bicarbonate of soda, mustard seeds, turmeric and more cold water to form a smooth batter – up to 1½ cups (375 ml). Set aside.

2. Steam the sweet potato or microwave it on high until tender.

3. Heat the olive oil in a large frying pan over medium heat, add the onion and mustard seeds and cook, stirring, until the onion is soft and golden and the mustard seeds start to pop. Add the chilli, garlic, ginger, turmeric and sweet potato and mix well over low heat for less than 5 minutes, until the garlic and ginger are cooked and the mixture is well combined. Set aside in a bowl. Cover to keep warm.

4. Wipe out the same frying pan and lightly spray with olive oil on medium heat, and pour the chickpea batter (enough to thinly coat the base of the frypan) into the pan for the first pancake. Tilt the pan to spread it out evenly over the base, and cook for a couple of minutes or until bubbles start to appear on the surface. Flip it over and cook for another couple of minutes until golden and cooked through. Remove and keep warm while you make the remaining

pancakes. You should have enough batter to make 4 pancakes in total.

5. Serve the pancakes with the spiced sweet potato and some Greek yoghurt.

SWEET POTATO CHILLI CON CARNE

Spice this up or down to suit your taste, but take my advice and make a double batch. It's a great one to heat up to have for lunch the following few days, and freezes well for an easy weeknight meal when you don't have time to cook something from scratch.

Serves 4

3 small sweet potatoes, peeled if desired
2 tablespoons olive oil
1 tablespoon Cajun spice mix
dried chilli flakes, to taste
dried oregano, to taste
1 brown onion, finely chopped
1 red capsicum, seeds and membrane removed, diced
1 x 400 g tin red kidney beans, drained and rinsed
1 tablespoon low-sodium tomato paste
160 g roma tomatoes or similar, roughly chopped/diced
flat-leaf parsley leaves, to garnish

1. Preheat the oven to 200°C and line a baking dish with baking paper.
2. Place the sweet potato in the prepared dish. Drizzle with 1 tablespoon olive oil and sprinkle the Cajun spice mix, chilli flakes and oregano over the top. Bake for 30 minutes or until tender. Remove and set aside to cool slightly.

3. Meanwhile, heat the remaining olive oil in a frying pan over medium heat, add the onion and capsicum and cook, stirring, for 5 minutes. Add the kidney beans, tomato paste, tomatoes, and 1 cup (250 ml) water. Bring to the boil, then reduce the heat and simmer for 10 minutes or until thickened.

4. When the sweet potato is cool enough to handle, cut it into small cubes and add it to the bean mixture. Garnish with parsley and serve.

BUTTERNUT PUMPKIN PIZZA

This is an exceptionally fun dish to make and one of my favourites! The pumpkin base adds a lot of flavour to the traditional pizza base. Topping your pizza with plenty of vegetables, rather than processed meats and cheese, is a good way to keep both fat and salt levels down, while at the same time increasing your fibre and vegetable intake. Use a low-fat shredded cheddar cheese for the topping; a light sprinkle is enough to bind all the ingredients.

Serves 4

500 g butternut pumpkin, peeled and cut into small pieces
3 cups (480 g) self-raising wholemeal flour
1½ tablespoons olive oil
low-sodium tomato paste
large handful of shredded cheddar cheese
250 g cherry or grape tomatoes, halved
small handful of snow peas, cut into small pieces
large handful of basil leaves

1. Preheat the oven to 200°C and line a large pizza tray with baking paper.
2. Steam the pumpkin for 5–10 minutes or until tender. Remove and allow to cool slightly.
3. Transfer pumpkin, flour and olive oil to a food processor/ blender and pulse until it just combines.

4. Scoop out the mixture onto a floured surface and knead for 5 minutes or until a smooth dough forms. It may still be a bit sticky, but this is fine. Place the dough on a plate, cover with plastic wrap and leave for 15 minutes.

5. Roll out the pizza dough and place on the prepared tray. (If you only have smaller trays, just make two pizzas.)

6. Spread the tomato paste over the base and sprinkle with half the cheese, then top with the tomatoes, snow peas and half the basil. Sprinkle evenly with the remaining cheese.

7. Bake for 20 minutes or until the cheese has melted and the base is cooked through. Test the dough, if you like, by sticking a fork into it – it should come out dry and clean.

8. Scatter the remaining basil over the pizza and serve hot.

Tip: To make your own self-raising flour, add 1½ teaspoons baking powder for every cup (160 g) of plain flour and sift together thoroughly.

BAKED FALAFEL

The traditional way to cook falafel is to deep-fry them, which can make them very high in energy due to the oil content. This healthy alternative is packed full of flavour and goodness, and is very satiating, helping you feel full for longer. From a nutritional point of view, it's better to use soaked, dried chickpeas but if you are short on time, 3 cups of rinsed, drained chickpeas would be the next best thing.

Serves 4

1 cup (200 g) dried chickpeas
large handful of flat-leaf parsley leaves
small handful of coriander leaves
small handful of dill leaves
1½ tablespoons olive oil
3 garlic cloves
1 tablespoon tahini or sesame seeds
1 teaspoon freshly ground black pepper
1 teaspoon ground cumin
pinch of cayenne pepper
Greek yoghurt, to serve
Greek salad (see page 131), to serve

1. Soak the chickpeas in a large bowl of water overnight. Drain well and spread out on a tea towel to air dry.
2. Place the parsley, coriander, dill and olive oil in a food processor (or blender) and mix until finely chopped.

3. Add the chickpeas, garlic, tahini or sesame seeds, pepper, cumin and cayenne pepper and blend until well combined. Gradually add small quantities of water if the processor is struggling to mix the ingredients.

4. Transfer the falafel mixture to a large bowl and cover tightly with plastic wrap. Refrigerate for at least 30 minutes; preferably, for up to 2 hours.

5. Preheat the oven to 180°C and line a baking tray with baking paper.

6. With wet hands, shape heaped tablespoons of the falafel into balls and place on the prepared tray.

7. Bake for 20 minutes or until golden and cooked through. Serve hot with Greek yoghurt and salad.

JAPANESE-INSPIRED SALMON

This method of cooking fish in foil is great, as the salmon retains its natural oils, preventing it from drying out, and meaning you don't need to add any oil. All the goodness and flavour are kept within the foil parcel, resulting in gently cooked, succulent fish.

Serves 4

4 Tasmanian salmon fillets, with skin
2 teaspoons wholegrain mustard
2 teaspoons white miso paste
blanched green vegetables or salad, to serve

1. Place the salmon fillets in a glass bowl. Smear the mustard and miso paste all over the fish, except for the skin. Cover with plastic wrap and marinate in the fridge for 10–30 minutes.
2. Preheat the oven to 180°C.
3. Remove the fish from the fridge and wrap each piece individually in foil. Place on a baking tray in a single layer and bake for 15 minutes. Check that it's cooked through – the precise cooking time can vary, depending on the size of the fillet.
4. Remove the parcels from the oven, and serve with blanched greens or a fresh salad.

VEGETARIAN LETTUCE CUPS

If you have time, dried lentils are better than tinned, but it is important to presoak them for this particular recipe. Just put 200 g dried lentils in a bowl, pour in enough water to cover them by 5 cm and soak overnight. While I love the flavour and texture the lentils bring to these lettuce cups, you can leave them out if you prefer – the dish will still be delicious.

Makes 8

3 tablespoons olive oil
4 large portobello mushrooms, finely chopped
2 small carrots, finely chopped
3 spring onions, finely chopped
1 x 400 g tin brown lentils (with no added salt), drained
small handful of flat-leaf parsley, finely chopped
1 red chilli, finely chopped (take the seeds out if you like)
1 garlic clove, crushed
1 tablespoon grated ginger
3 tablespoons soy sauce
⅓ cup (45 g) crushed unsalted peanuts
1 iceberg lettuce
bean sprouts, to serve

1. Heat 2 tablespoons olive oil in a large frying pan or wok over high heat, add the mushrooms and cook for 2 minutes or until softened. Remove and set aside.

2. Heat the remaining oil in the pan, add the carrots and spring onions and cook for 2 minutes. Mix in the drained lentils.

3. Add the parsley, chilli, garlic and ginger and cook for a further 2 minutes, then pour in the soy sauce and cook for 2 minutes, tossing in the mushrooms to coat. Mix in the peanuts.

4. Break off 8 good-sized leaves from the core of the lettuce to make individual cups. Spoon the mushroom filling into the lettuce cups and sprinkle the bean sprouts over the top. Enjoy while they're hot.

SALMON RISSOLES

This is such a versatile meal, making it an excellent standby for a quick weeknight dinner. You can use sweet potatoes instead of regular potatoes, if that's what you happen to have. Frozen vegetables are another great alternative – again, they are snap frozen at the time of picking, so often retain most, if not all, of their nutritional value. They can also be bought in individual mixed bags, making preparation easy, so I encourage you to keep a supply in your freezer.

Makes 12

6 potatoes, peeled, roughly chopped
1 red onion, diced
1 x 210 g tin red salmon (with no added salt), drained
1 egg, lightly beaten
1 cup (100 g) dried breadcrumbs
olive oil spray
fresh salad or blanched vegetables, to serve

1. Place the potatoes in a saucepan of cold water, bring to the boil, and cook for 5–10 minutes, or until tender but not overly soft. At about 5 minutes, add the onion to the pan.
2. Drain the onion and potatoes and mash them well. Mix through the salmon, then form the mixture into 12 evenly sized patties.
3. Dip the patties into the beaten egg, allowing any excess to drain off, then coat them all over with the breadcrumbs.

4. Spray a large frying pan with olive oil and heat over low heat. Add the patties and cook for 5 minutes or until golden brown on both sides.

5. Serve with a side salad or your choice of vegetables.

PUMPKIN AND LENTIL CURRY

This is a quick and simple curry utilising many of the store cupboard essentials that you should have in stock. The herbs and spices bring out the flavour and texture. The pumpkin can be replaced with sweet potato or with potato, if preferred.

Serves 4

1 tablespoon olive oil

1 teaspoon ground cumin

½ teaspoon ground turmeric

1 garlic clove, crushed

2 cups (230 g) butternut pumpkin, peeled and cut into
   approximately 2 cm diced pieces

1 x 400 g tin lentils (preferably brown lentils), (no added salt
   variety)

1 x 400 g tin tomatoes (no added salt variety)

120 g basmati or doongara rice

coriander leaves, to garnish

1. Heat the olive oil in a large deep frying pan over medium heat. Add the cumin, turmeric and garlic and cook for 2 minutes or until fragrant.

2. Stir in the diced pumpkin, lentils and tomatoes, and combine well. Reduce the heat to low, then cover and simmer for 30 minutes or until the pumpkin is cooked through.

3. Meanwhile, cook the rice until it's fluffy and tender (see next page, 'How to cook rice').

4. Divide the rice and curry among four plates or bowls and garnish with fresh coriander leaves.

HOW TO COOK RICE

To prevent your rice from becoming gluggy, use one of the following methods. As a general rule, brown rice takes approximately twice as long to cook as white rice. For each of the below cooking methods, you can try adding stock to the rice for extra flavour. This would replace the water specified for each method.

1. Absorption. This method requires 1½ cups (375 ml) water for every cup (200 g) uncooked rice. Combine the rice and water in a saucepan and bring to the boil, stirring occasionally. Reduce the heat and simmer, covered, for 12–15 minutes or until tender.
2. Microwave. This method requires 2 cups (500 ml) hot water for every cup (200 g) uncooked rice. Combine the rice and water in a large microwave-safe dish with a lid and microwave on high power, stirring occasionally, for 10–12 minutes or until tender.
3. Boil. This method requires 1.5–2 litres water for every cup (200 g) uncooked rice. Bring the water to the boil in a large saucepan. Add the rice and stir until the water comes back to the boil. Reduce the heat to medium–high and boil, uncovered, for 12–15 minutes or until the rice is tender.

SNACKS AND SIDES

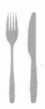

BEETROOT DIP

I like to serve this attractive-looking dip with baked wholemeal Lebanese bread. Drizzle a very small quantity of olive oil over the bread and scatter some fresh rosemary leaves over the top. Bake in an oven at 180 degrees Celsius for a few minutes until crisp and lightly golden. Break up the bread and serve with the dip.

Makes 2 cups

500 g (about 3 medium) beetroot
1 garlic clove, crushed
200 g no-fat or low-fat natural yoghurt
1 teaspoon ground cumin
2 teaspoons lemon juice

1. Place the beetroot in a large saucepan, cover with water and bring to the boil. Cook for about 30 minutes or until tender (test with a skewer – it should go through easily).
2. Remove the beetroot and set aside to cool for a few minutes. Peel them while they are still warm and roughly chop.
3. Blend the beetroot, garlic, yoghurt, cumin and lemon juice until smooth and well combined.
4. Serve with wholemeal Lebanese bread or your choice of vegetable dippers.

BEETROOT HUMMUS

Both the beetroot dip and this beetroot hummus are huge hits when entertaining crowds. Double the quantities so you have some leftovers for yourself – the dip and hummus make a great snack with vegetable sticks, such as carrot and celery, or strips of toasted wholegrain bread.

Makes 2 cups

450 g (about 3 small) beetroot
1 x 420 g tin chickpeas, drained and rinsed
2 garlic cloves, crushed
1 tablespoon tahini
1 tablespoon lemon juice
3 tablespoons olive oil

1. Place the beetroot in a large saucepan, cover with water and bring to the boil. Cook for about 30 minutes or until tender (test with a skewer – it should go through easily).
2. Remove the beetroot and set aside to cool for a few minutes. Peel them while they are still warm and roughly chop.
3. Blend the beetroot, chickpeas, garlic, tahini and lemon juice until well combined. You might want to add the ingredients gradually, along with splashes of water to achieve the right consistency. Finally, gradually blend in the olive oil until the mixture is thick and smooth.

4. Serve with your choice of vegetable dippers or strips of wholegrain toast.

ROASTED CAPSICUMS

These smoky flavoured capsicums are a great entrée when entertaining guests. It's well worth investing in some stainless steel skewers, as they are efficient conductors of heat and great for the barbecue. They also save you the hassle of having to pre-soak bamboo skewers, which you should always do before cooking so they don't burn.

Serves 4

2 green capsicums, halved, seeds and membrane removed
2 red capsicums, halved, seeds and membrane removed
3 tablespoons olive oil
2 small garlic cloves, crushed
1 tablespoon chopped flat-leaf parsley

1. Preheat the oven to 180°C. If you are using bamboo or wooden skewers, soak them in water for about 20 minutes before threading on the ingredients.
2. Place the capsicum halves, skin-side-up, on a baking tray and roast for 3–5 minutes or until the skin is slightly blackened and blistered. Set aside until cool enough to handle, then remove the skin and cut the flesh into bite-sized pieces.
3. Combine the olive oil, garlic and parsley in a bowl, add the capsicum and coat it. Allow it to stand for 5–10 minutes.
4. Thread the capsicum pieces onto skewers, then lightly grill in a pre-heated chargrill pan for 3 minutes to warm, and serve.

SPICY CHICKEN BITES WITH TOMATO SALSA

These chicken bites are a great snack on their own, but I find them particularly moreish with a freshly made tomato salsa. You can make the salsa while the chicken is cooking and enjoy it still warm from the pan, although it can also be enjoyed cool.

Serves 6

400 g chicken breast fillets, cut into bite-sized pieces
4 egg whites
dried breadcrumbs, to coat (100 g should be plenty)
dried chilli flakes, to taste

Tomato salsa
250 g cherry or grape tomatoes
2 spring onions, finely chopped
2 tablespoons sweet chilli sauce
2 tablespoons finely chopped coriander

1. Preheat the oven to 200°C and line a baking tray with baking paper.
2. Whisk the egg whites in a shallow bowl. Combine the breadcrumbs and chilli flakes in another bowl.
3. Toss the chicken pieces in the egg white, allowing any excess to drip off, then toss in the breadcrumbs and chilli flakes until well coated.

4. Arrange the chicken pieces in a single layer on the prepared tray and bake for 12 minutes or until cooked through.

5. Meanwhile, to make the salsa, place the tomatoes and spring onions in a small saucepan and cook over low heat for a few minutes or until the spring onions have softened and the tomatoes have started to collapse. Stir in the sweet chilli sauce and simmer for 1 minute, then remove from heat and stir in the coriander. Allow to cool for a few minutes.

6. Serve the chicken straight from the oven with the tomato salsa.

TOMATO, ROSEMARY AND CARAMELISED ONION MINI PIZZAS

Rosemary is easy to grow and very low maintenance, so it will survive during those times when you are away from home or have become a little lax towards your gardening responsibilities. Its earthy flavour makes a wonderful addition to many foods, including these pizzas. You could use grape or cherry tomatoes instead, if you prefer – you'll need about three punnets. If you are having the pizzas as a light lunch, it would serve four people, but you could also offer them as a nibble with drinks.

Makes 12

2 pizza bases (fresh or frozen)
8 ripe tomatoes, halved
dried chilli flakes, to taste
2 tablespoons olive oil
4 red onions, thinly sliced
4 garlic cloves, crushed
4 sprigs rosemary, leaves stripped
½ cup (140 g) low-sodium tomato paste

1. Preheat the oven to 180°C. Line a baking tray with baking paper.
2. Cut each pizza base into six small circles.

3. Place the tomato halves, cut side up, on a baking tray, sprinkle with the chilli flakes and roast for 15 minutes or until soft.

4. Meanwhile, heat the olive oil in a large saucepan over low heat, add the onion, garlic and about two-thirds of the rosemary leaves and cook for around 20 minutes, or until the onion is soft and caramelised.

5. Spread the tomato paste over the mini pizza bases and top with the caramelised onion and roast tomato. Sprinkle the remaining rosemary over the top and bake for 10–15 minutes or until the bases are cooked through. Serve hot.

GREEK-STYLE LAMB SLIDERS

These delicious mini burgers are a fun meal to cook as a family. Lamb is a wonderful way to add variety to the weekly menu.

Makes 12

2 teaspoons olive oil
2 garlic cloves, crushed
2 teaspoons ground cumin
2 tablespoons lemon juice
500 g lamb mince (lean variety)
1 egg
sprinkle of wholemeal plain flour (optional)
olive oil spray
12 mini burger buns (preferably wholemeal)
avocado
2 tomatoes, sliced
rocket or baby spinach leaves, to serve

1. Combine the olive oil, garlic, cumin and lemon juice in a large bowl. Add the lamb mince and egg and, with clean hands, mix thoroughly. Add a tiny sprinkle of flour if the mixture is a little wet, then form it into 12 evenly sized patties.
2. Transfer the patties to a plate and cover with plastic wrap. Leave in the fridge for 10–30 minutes.

3. Heat a barbecue grill, cast-iron grill plate or heavy frying pan over low heat and spray with olive oil. Add the patties and cook, turning once, for 5–7 minutes or until cooked through (no pink should be evident).

4. Toast the rolls if you like, then spread the base of each with a thin layer of avocado. Add the patties, tomatoes and a little rocket or spinach, and serve.

Tip: Minced (or ground) meat implies that the surface and the interior of the meat have been mixed. This means the meat may be fully contaminated with bacteria and must be entirely cooked through so there is not even a hint of pink in the cooked patties.

MOROCCAN CHICKEN RICE PAPER ROLLS WITH PEANUT SAUCE

This is a terrific recipe for when you want to get children in the kitchen – they love choosing the fillings and rolling up their own creations. Leftover cucumber, capsicum and carrot can be chopped up and kept in the fridge as snacks – vegetable sticks go perfectly with the beetroot dip and beetroot hummus on pages 167 and 168.

Makes 6–8

250 g lean chicken mince

1 garlic clove, crushed

½ teaspoon grated ginger

1 teaspoon Moroccan seasoning (optional)

1 tablespoon olive oil

20 g rice vermicelli (you only need a small handful of noodles)

6–8 rice paper wrappers

2 small carrots, cut into matchsticks

½ capsicum, seeds and membrane removed, cut into matchsticks

½ continental cucumber, cut into matchsticks

bean sprouts, to serve

small handful of crushed peanuts

Peanut sauce

1 teaspoon olive oil

1 garlic clove, crushed

1 small red chilli, finely chopped

3 tablespoons natural peanut butter (100% peanuts)

1 tablespoon lemon juice

1. To make the peanut sauce, heat the olive oil in a small saucepan over medium heat. Add the garlic and chilli and cook for 1 minute. Add the peanut butter, then reduce the heat to low and cook, stirring well, as you add the lemon juice and ½ cup (125 ml) water. Continue to stir and cook for 3–5 minutes or until the sauce has thickened. Cover and keep warm while you prepare the rice paper rolls.
2. Place the chicken mince, garlic, ginger and Moroccan seasoning (if using) in a bowl and mix well.
3. Heat the olive oil in a frying pan over low heat, add the mince and cook for 5 minutes, stirring regularly and breaking up any lumps with a wooden spoon. Remove from the heat.
4. Meanwhile, place the vermicelli noodles in a heatproof bowl, cover with boiling water and leave for 2 minutes or until softened. Drain well.
5. Working with one rice paper wrapper at a time, dip into hot water for 30 seconds, then place on a moist tea towel and wait until it softens.
6. Spread a small amount of chicken, vermicelli, carrot, capsicum, cucumber and bean sprouts on one end of the wrapper and sprinkle with a few peanuts. Fold the bottom edge over the filling, then fold in both sides and roll up to form the rice paper roll. Repeat with the remaining wrappers and filling.
7. Serve the rice paper rolls with the peanut sauce for dipping.

ROSEMARY AND THYME-INFUSED ROASTED VEGETABLES

This is a great option for an evening meal when you don't feel like having anything too extravagant. It's a simple way of getting plenty of vitamins and minerals, while at the same time clearing out any vegetables languishing in the crisper drawer. I don't give any quantities, as you can make as much or as little as you like.

vegetables, such as broccoli, cauliflower, sweet potato, carrot
   and capsicum
olive oil, for drizzling
rosemary and thyme leaves

1. Preheat the oven to 180°C and line a roasting tin with baking paper.
2. Cut the vegetables into evenly sized pieces and place in the prepared tin. Drizzle with olive oil and scatter rosemary and thyme leaves over the top, then toss gently to coat thoroughly with the herbs and oil.
3. Roast for 20–30 minutes or until all the vegetables are tender and cooked through. The cooking time may vary, depending on which vegetables you use and how large the pieces are.

CRUNCHY ROSEMARY POTATO WEDGES

These always seem to disappear the minute I put them on the table, and I'm not surprised. Who doesn't love crisp, golden potato wedges? For best results, cut the potatoes into similar-sized pieces to ensure even cooking. Starchy potatoes of the coliban variety tend to be the best for baking.

Serves 6

2 teaspoons mixed dried herbs

1 tablespoon rosemary leaves

1 teaspoon hot paprika

½ teaspoon salt

2 tablespoons olive oil

1 kg potatoes, cut into evenly sized wedges

1. Preheat the oven to 220°C and line a baking tray or flat pizza tray with baking paper.
2. Place the mixed herbs, rosemary, paprika, salt and olive oil in a large ziplock bag and shake to combine.
3. Add the potato wedges to the bag and shake to coat evenly with the herb oil.
4. Arrange the wedges on the prepared tray in a single layer and bake, turning once or twice, for 20–30 minutes or until crisp and golden. Serve hot!

'THE BROTHERS' LOAF

This is something that was one of my family's favourites, as we would make more than one loaf at a time and use them as a wholesome and filling snack through the week. Since it is quite dense, a small piece is more than enough at one sitting. The loaf keeps well in the fridge, so make it at the weekend, when you have a little time, and enjoy it through the week. It's also delicious toasted. There are endless variations on this recipe – my family makes at least a dozen different versions, and I encourage you to experiment too. Try adding other ingredients, such as chia seeds, or using hazelnuts and/or walnuts in place of the almonds.

Makes 1 large loaf

5 large eggs (or 6 small ones), separated
250 g almonds
50 g dried chickpeas
5 bananas, mashed
125 g honey

1. Line a large loaf tin with baking paper. There is no need to pre-heat the oven.
2. Whisk the egg whites in a clean bowl until soft peaks form.
3. Using a high-powered blender, blend the almonds and chickpeas to a fine consistency (powder).

4. Using an electric mixer, combine the almond mixture, banana, honey and egg yolks to form a smooth batter. Gently fold in the egg whites.

5. Pour the batter into the prepared tin and place in a cold oven. Set the temperature to 160°C and bake for 1 to 1½ hours or until a skewer inserted in the centre comes out clean.

6. Turn the loaf out onto a wire rack and cool for 30 minutes before slicing.

SWEET AND SAVOURY TREATS

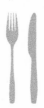

POMEGRANATE AND DARK CHOCOLATE BARK

Many people avoid pomegranates because they are unsure how to eat them. They can also be messy, as the seeds are trapped by membranes within the fruit and must be removed. Picking them out with your fingers creates a big mess (trust me on this) and I've discovered the best way to extract them is under water. Cut the pomegranate into quarters and place in a large bowl of cold water. Rub the fruit under water with your thumbs until the kernels pop out and sink to the bottom and the white membrane floats to the top. Now you just drain off the water and membrane and you are left with the beautiful seeds.

Serves 6

200 g dark chocolate (make sure it contains at least 70% cocoa), broken into pieces
large handful of rolled oats
large handful of unsalted raw cashews, crushed
seeds of ½ pomegranate

1. Preheat the oven to 120°C and line a deep baking tray with baking paper.
2. Scatter the chocolate over the prepared tray and place in the oven to melt (this will only take a few minutes).
3. Remove the tray and spread the chocolate evenly over the baking paper with the back of a spoon. Sprinkle the oats, cashews and pomegranate seeds over the chocolate.

4. Set aside to cool for 10 minutes and place in the fridge for 30 minutes to set.

5. Remove the bark from the baking paper and break into pieces to serve.

CARROT CAKE SLICE

There are only a few ingredients in this delicious slice, so they need to be good quality. Vanilla adds a warm sweetness to baked goods but I do urge you to buy extract rather than the cheaper essence. The difference between the two is that essence is a chemically developed flavouring, while extract comes straight from the vanilla bean. In my view, there really is no contest.

Makes 2 cakes, which serve 12 people

300 g almonds
3 small–medium carrots
3 eggs
2 teaspoons vanilla extract
3 teaspoons dried cinnamon
2½ teaspoons baking powder
1 cup (130 g) dried cranberries
3 tablespoons olive oil
160 ml maple syrup (or use honey)

1. Preheat the oven to 160°C and line two baking trays with baking paper.
2. Place the almonds in a high-powered blender and blend to a fine consistency (powder). You can use almond meal instead, which means you could skip this step.

3. Grate the carrots into a large bowl and add the ground almonds, eggs, vanilla, cinnamon, baking powder, cranberries, olive oil and maple syrup. Mix thoroughly.

4. Pour the batter evenly into the prepared trays and bake for 30–40 minutes or until cooked through.

5. Allow to cool completely on wire racks before cutting into slices to serve.

BUTTERNUT PUMPKIN AND OAT SCONES

This recipe is a perfect pairing of maple syrup and pumpkin, resulting in a deliciously nutritious snack that is perfect when entertaining guests. These scones are best enjoyed with a spread, such as whole-fruit jam.

Makes 10

260 g peeled butternut pumpkin, cut into small pieces
230 g wholemeal self-raising flour, plus extra for dipping
1 teaspoon baking powder
½ teaspoon ground cinnamon
1 tablespoon maple syrup
3 tablespoons (60 ml) olive oil
rolled oats, for coating

1. Preheat the oven to 180°C and line a large baking tray with baking paper.
2. Boil or steam pumpkin until tender, then set aside to cool.
3. Mix the flour, baking powder and cinnamon in a bowl.
4. Place the maple syrup, olive oil and cooled pumpkin in a separate bowl and mash until smooth and well mixed.
5. Add the pumpkin mixture to the dry ingredients and work them together with your hands to form a soft dough.
6. Spread a thin layer of rolled oats over a large chopping board. Roll out the pumpkin dough on top of the oats to a thickness of about 3 cm, then sprinkle some more oats over the top.

7. Dip an egg cup or small biscuit cutter in flour to prevent it from sticking to the dough. Cut out 10 scones and place them on the baking tray, gently gathering the dough together and rerolling it if necessary. Space the scones slightly apart on the prepared tray and bake for 25–30 minutes or until risen and lightly golden.

8. Allow the scones to cool on wire racks; they can be wrapped in a tea towel while cooling if you prefer a softer crust. Serve slightly warm.

Tip: Olive oil can be used for all methods of cooking (except deep-frying, which you won't be doing anyway), and should be substituted if other oils are recommended in recipes. Just make sure that the heat is not too high, as this will cause the oil to smoke in the pan. If the oil smokes, it has turned rancid, and you must clean the pan and start again.

GRILLED PAPAYA, PINEAPPLE AND PEAR SKEWERS

This is a fun snack for children to help prepare. Of course, a fresh fruit salad without the added condiments is better still and may be enjoyed every day but it's important to try to curb any potential 'comfort' eating with a sweet food that is also very healthy. These skewers fit the bill.

Makes 6

3 tablespoons brown sugar
2 cm piece of ginger, peeled and sliced
1 ripe pear, cut into bite-sized pieces
½ ripe pineapple, cut into bite-sized pieces
½ ripe papaya, cut into bite-sized pieces

1. If you are using bamboo or wooden skewers, soak them in water for about 20 minutes before threading on the ingredients. This will stop them burning during cooking.
2. Combine the sugar, ginger and 3 tablespoons of water in a saucepan and simmer over medium heat for 3 minutes or until the sugar has dissolved. Remove from heat and allow to cool, then strain into a cup.
3. Thread the fruit onto the skewers and brush lightly with the ginger syrup.
4. Heat a barbecue grill, cast-iron hot plate or frying pan over high heat. Lower to medium heat and add the skewers, cooking for 2 minutes on each side or until lightly browned. Brush again with ginger syrup and serve.

REFERENCES

1 http://www.aihw.gov.au/overweight-and-obesity/

2 http://www.abs.gov.au/ausstats/abs@.nsf/Products/ B2B67E82EFA3EB2ACA25789C0023DAB9?open document

3 http://www.nejm.org/doi/full/10.1056/nejmoa1105816

4 http://www.thelancet.com/journals/landia/article/ PIIS2213-8587(14)70200-1/abstract

5 https://www.ncbi.nlm.nih.gov/pmc/articles/ PMC4443883/

6 http://www.nejm.org/doi/full/10.1056/ NEJMoa0804748

7 https://www.ncbi.nlm.nih.gov/pubmed/20182054

8 www.sampletemplates.com/business-templates/urine-color-chart.html

9 http://www.nhmrc.gov.au/_files_nhmrc/publications/ attachments/ds10-alcohol.pdf

ACKNOWLEDGEMENTS

You must wait for that which you seek. Challenge yourself and surround yourself with those who challenge you, and who devote their love to you, as you would to them.

To my mother, Diane; my brother, Andrew; and my fiancée, Sally. I am very grateful for all that you have done for me, now and for eternity.

To all my friends who have supported this journey in writing a book, thank you for the many comments on each version.

To all those patients I have come across on my professional journey: this book would never have been possible without you, and I hope my Interval Weight Loss plan will go on to help many more people in need of guidance.

WEIGHT-LOSS TEMPLATE

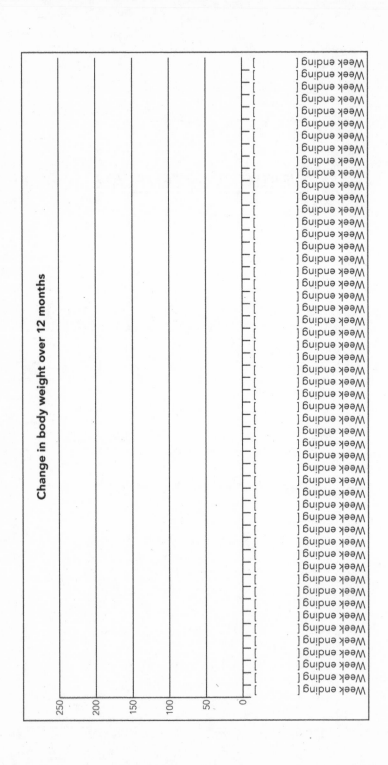

RECIPE INDEX

GENERAL INDEX